THE HERBAL
MEDICINE COOKBOOK

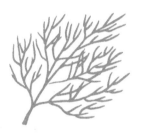

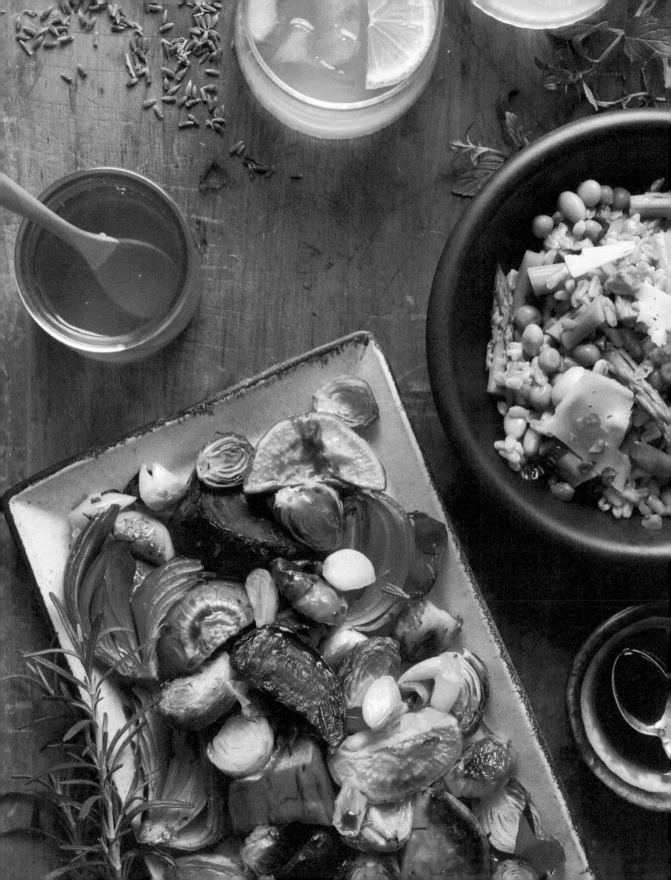

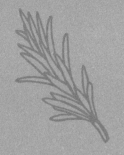

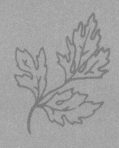

THE HERBAL MEDICINE COOKBOOK

Everyday Recipes to Boost Your Health

SUSAN HESS AND TINA SAMS

PHOTOGRAPHY BY EVI ABELER

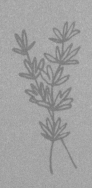

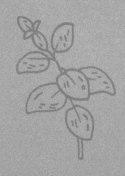

R
ROCKRIDGE
PRESS

For general information on our other products and services or to obtain technical support, please contact our Customer Care Department within the U.S. at (866) 744-2665, or outside the U.S. at (510) 253-0500.

Rockridge Press publishes its books in a variety of electronic and print formats. Some content that appears in print may not be available in electronic books, and vice versa.

Interior Designer: Jess Morphew
Cover Designer: Katy Brown
Photo Art Director / Art Manager: Karen Beard
Editor: Vanessa Ta
Production Editor: Erum Khan
Photography © 2018 Evi Abeler, food styling by Albane Sharrard
Author photo © Donna Connor
Illustration © shooarts/Shutterstock

ISBN: Print 978-1-64152-264-9 | eBook 978-1-64152-265-6

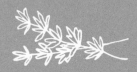

FOR EMILY & RILEY,
WHO MOVED ME
TO FEED YOU,
BUT TRUSTED ME
TO NOURISH YOU.

CONTENTS

INTRODUCTION IX

PART ONE

HERBAL MEDICINE

PART TWO

RECIPES

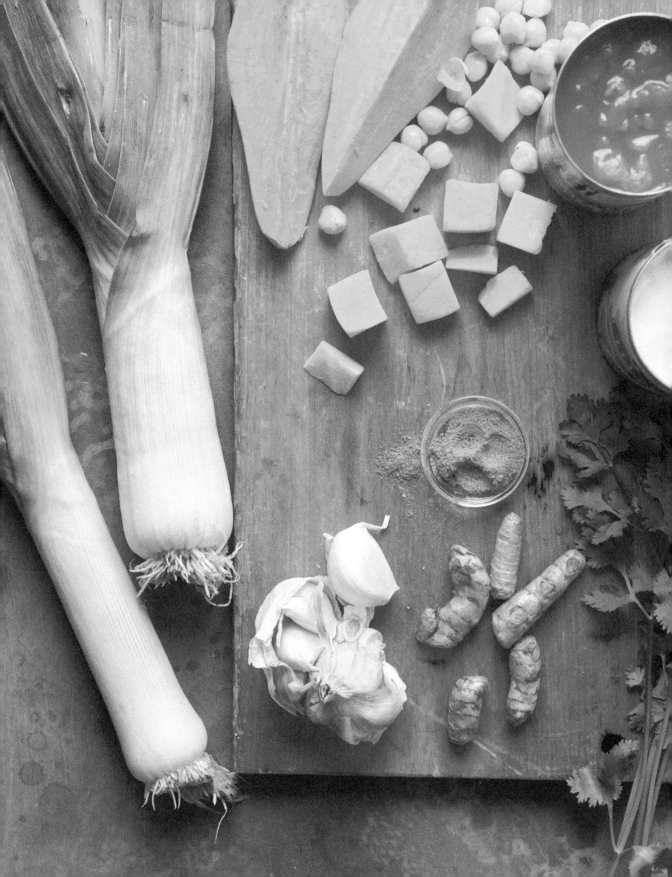

INTRODUCTION

Nearly 40 years ago, I wandered into my neighbor Peggy's garden for the first time. It was alive and overflowing with colorful vegetables, fragrant herbs, and flowers. Her two small children danced through it like butterflies, nibbling cherry tomatoes and sipping fresh chamomile tea from tiny bowls. Inside, Peggy's kitchen held her own handwoven baskets laden with vegetables, aromatic herbs hung to dry, and a spicy concoction simmering on the stove. In a single visit, I observed how fresh foods, pungent herbs, aromatic cooking, and healthy, vibrant children seemed naturally, almost magically, connected and inseparable. It was my first taste of a natural holistic lifestyle with a kitchen at its hub. Peggy took everyday life skills, like gardening, cooking, and raising healthy children, and elevated them to an art form in my young eyes.

When I decided to put up jars of peaches that summer, with no idea how, I spontaneously bought an entire bushel, drove home, and then called my grandmother to ask her what to do next. She got in her car and drove 40 miles wearing an apron to show me. We canned 15 quarts of peaches that afternoon. It impressed upon me the value of passing on skills centered in the kitchen. My grandmother and my mother had both dedicated their lives to the nursing profession. With the birth of my own children, it seemed inevitable that a deep-rooted interest in healing would soon be stirring in myself, as well.

When my three-year-old developed a cough that turned into pneumonia, many trips to the doctor ensued. After two rounds of antibiotics and a hospital stay looming on the horizon, I felt helpless and scared. A local nurse came to our home to show me how to apply a mustard plaster to my son's chest. In the kitchen, while we ground pungent black mustard seeds and water into a paste, she hummed and lifted the lid to my own simmering soup pot. With a wink, she suggested that I add more garlic, which I amended. My son recovered rapidly, and I felt the desire to learn more. Much more.

Creating and maintaining health through the lens of the family kitchen and sharing this lifestyle with others is at the very heart of my life's work as an herbalist. I recognize the same hunger for healing knowledge in the eyes of every student I have the pleasure of sharing with. It's my pleasure to continue that tradition here on these pages with you.

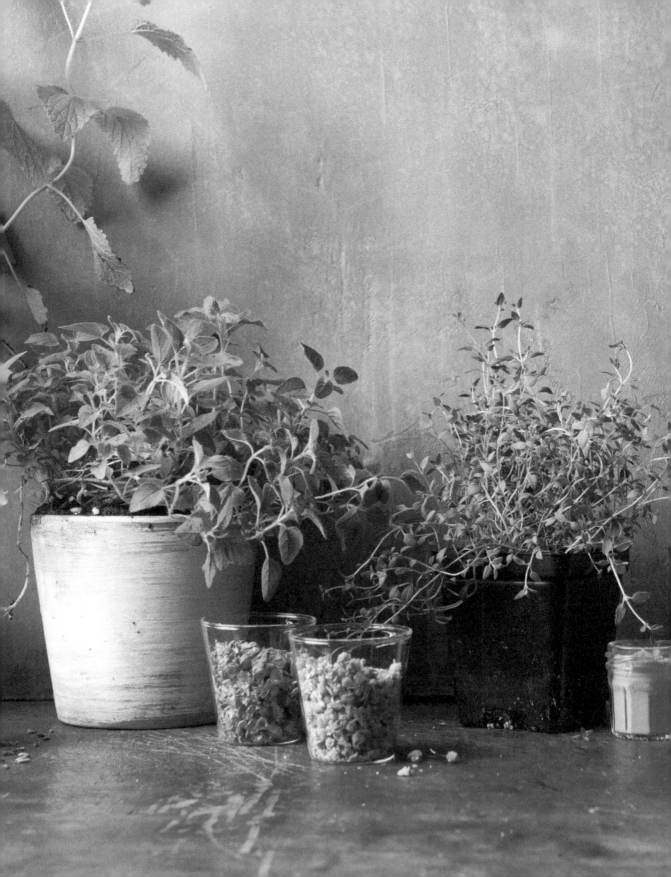

PART ONE

HERBAL MEDICINE

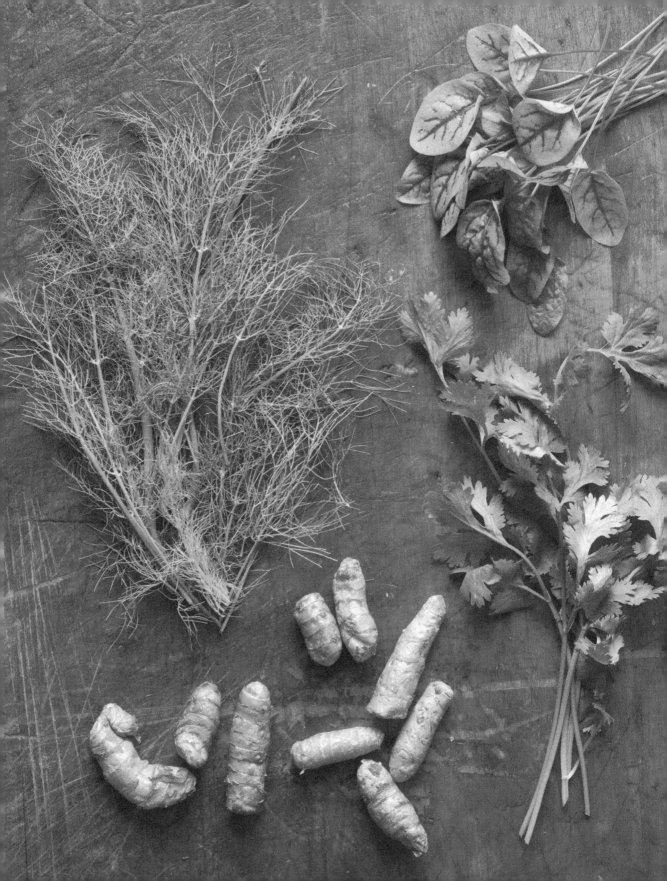

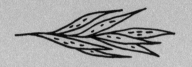

CHAPTER ONE

WHY COOK WITH HERBAL MEDICINE?

The humble domestic kitchen has been the epicenter of care and nourishment of body and soul for thousands of years. Imagine a time when there was no distinction between nourishing foods and healing medicines. By artfully and mindfully combining seasonal foods and medicinal herbs, we can support the body through illness. When this knowledge is passed on, it ensures the health and well-being of families, communities, and future generations. I can't think of a more meaningful and inspiring way to live!

I'm excited that you are here, in my own humble kitchen, ready to explore and embrace the basic concepts of everyday medicinal cooking. May you be inspired to create, enjoy, and above all, share these flavorful foods as an integral part of your holistic life.

HERBAL MEDICINE

It goes without saying that humans and plants have coexisted since the beginning of time. How they interacted was largely a mystery until 5,000 years ago, when several early civilizations began to document their native food and medicinal plant uses. Traditional Chinese and Ayurvedic practitioners were trained in diagnostic and healing techniques with centuries of tradition and philosophy behind them. All aspects of a person's vitality were observed for diagnosis and treatment, including not only the physical state but the health of the emotional, mental, and spiritual being, as well. Today, the World Health Organization estimates that between 65 and 80 percent of the world's population (5 to 6 billion people) still rely on some form of traditional plant-based medicine and healing foods as their primary form of health care.

Yet here in the United States, food choices and their connection to health may be somewhat overlooked as a valuable healing tool in a fractured mainstream health care system. Western medicine certainly excels at diagnostics, alleviating symptoms, and fighting disease. But learning to bridge the wide gap between Western health care and personal preventive health care based on a natural lifestyle with healthy choices in foods and herbs is an idea that many can embrace and obtain. The recipes in this book provide you with a great start to making that a reality.

WHAT IS A MEDICINAL HERB?

When people first consider how they might use medicinal herbs in the kitchen, they probably think about making a cup of tea to ease a sore throat, to help digest a large meal, or as a way to relax before bed. Medicinal teas are generally pleasant tasting, sipped, savored, and enjoyed at the end of a long day or shared with a friend. That sounds like the start of some good medicine right there, doesn't it?

Learning how to take a step or two beyond tea-making to incorporate culinary herbs and spices into everyday foods can be a seamless way to enjoy new tastes and build optimal health and balance. What does "balance" mean in relation to the body? Balance simply means encouraging a gentle shift from average health to peak health using medicinal cooking. Using herbs and spices in everyday foods is the one of the easiest, most economical, and most flavorful ways to achieve that goal. Small amounts of herbs and spices added to daily meals can aid the digestive process, stimulate metabolism or immune response, or help reduce inflammation. Most herbs and spices are incredibly high in antioxidants, which can help prevent degenerative disease states in aging.

THE POWER OF HERBS

It is important to mention that while herbs are generally considered gentle, natural, and safe, educating yourself about how they work in your body is a vital (and empowering) piece of your overall health plan. There is so much to learn about the gentle, but nuanced, power of herbs.

The recipes in this book will reintroduce you to familiar herbs and spices that you may already have in your garden or kitchen cabinet. You will also be introduced to how those familiar tastes can have gentle, positive effects on your health. Any possible safety concerns or drug interactions will be mentioned right up-front for those who have special health considerations.

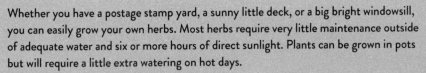

GROWING YOUR OWN HERBS

Whether you have a postage stamp yard, a sunny little deck, or a big bright windowsill, you can easily grow your own herbs. Most herbs require very little maintenance outside of adequate water and six or more hours of direct sunlight. Plants can be grown in pots but will require a little extra watering on hot days.

Annuals, such as basil, dill, or fennel, can easily be started by seed in the spring. Annuals grow rapidly throughout the summer and complete their life cycle in the fall. With a few small harvests per month, the plants will thrive and give you ample leaves to use fresh or to dry for the winter months. To keep basil growing strong, it is important to routinely pinch off the flowers.

Woody perennial herbs, like sage, thyme, oregano, and mint, are best purchased as small plants. They grow more slowly. Perennials can survive outside over the winter and live up to a few years. It is ideal to give them a pot or place in the garden with some room to grow. Perennials also benefit from a good pruning once or twice per year. Pruning (and using!) the top third of the plant will keep it growing lush and full!

The good news is that the herbs and spices added to the fruits, vegetables, and meats in these recipes are in amounts that simply awaken the body's systems in slow and gentle ways. Stimulating simple digestive function with carminative spices that encourage increased nutrient absorption alone will be a great and positive boon to your health. You will be happy with your newfound knowledge and kitchen skills, I promise!

THE TASTE OF HERBS

Learning about the medicinal uses of herbs is most certainly a lifelong study. Using culinary herbs and foods based on their tastes is, without a doubt, the first step and the very foundation of everyday medicinal cooking.

Simply discovering how an herb's taste activates the taste buds and creates a specific physiological reaction will also illustrate how that same taste can be used medicinally.

Most culinary herbs fall into five distinct taste categories, each with its own healing profile. Within each taste profile, there is a unique set of physiological qualities (such as warming, drying, cooling, or moistening) that are also associated with each herb. These five tastes, their qualities, and how they affect the body are often referred to as herbal "energetics."

The taste of herbs and spices immediately connects us to our own personal chemistry. Have you ever felt warmed from the inside after eating a slice of a cinnamon-laden apple pie? Or immediately cooled down by cucumber salad with mint? These specific tastes create physiological activities within our bodies that are experienced viscerally. No memorizing needed. With some observation and experimentation, learning to cook with herbs in this way might mean asking yourself: What pungent tea can I brew to take this bone-deep chill away? What could I prepare for dinner after a long, hot day in the sun? Once you get to know the five tastes of herbs and how they can help bring balance to your health, you might choose bitter greens to stimulate a sluggish digestion or reach for horseradish, ginger, and garlic when you feel a cold coming on. The five tastes are the foundation of medicinal cooking. Let's take a good look at these tastes, along with their associated qualities, and get to know some of the herbs in each category.

FURTHER STUDY: THE ENERGETICS OF HERBS

Further interest in the taste of herbs often leads to the topic of "energetics." In the simplest of terms, energetics is a system of categorizing herbs and foods based on their taste, temperature, and moisture and how that taste, temperature, and moisture can create physiological activity or change in the body.

Let's take a quick look at how energetic qualities are assigned to individual categories of herbs.

WARMING HERBS turn up metabolism, stimulate circulation, and increase warmth (in the case of cayenne) and energy. Herbs that have warm or hot activity are used to help fight off viruses and bacteria (garlic, lavender, or oregano), when the body has excess mucus (sage or thyme), or to aid digestion (cinnamon or ginger). Imagine building a fire in a cold room, drinking a cup of ginger tea on a cold day, or rubbing a warming liniment on cold, stiff joints.

COOLING HERBS slow down metabolism and decrease redness, heat, irritation, and inflammation in the body. Cooling herbs might soothe a sore throat (rose petal) or heartburn (chamomile). Imagine closing the damper on a woodstove, sticking your feet in a cold stream, or tasting a few bites of cool cucumber salad with a spicy, hot curry dish.

MOISTENING HERBS bring moisture and softness to dry, hard, or brittle tissues and are beneficial to dry conditions such as chronic constipation or excessively dry skin. There are relatively few culinary herbs that are moistening, so we will turn to foods that have moistening qualities, such as good-quality fats, oatmeal, barley, cooked apples and peaches, pears, bananas, winter squashes, and dairy products in small quantities. Astragalus and fennel tea would provide some moistening qualities, as well. Imagine sucking on a slippery elm lozenge when you have a dry throat, slathering moisturizer on winter skin, or soaking dried beans overnight.

DRYING HERBS relieve stagnant, swollen, fluid-filled tissues and remove excess moisture, such as mucus (sage or thyme), bringing the tissues back to firm and dense. Many common culinary herbs and spices have drying activity. Imagine allowing a plump, juicy mushroom to sit on a countertop for a few days or hanging heavy, wet laundry to dry on a sunny clothes line.

To gain a broader understanding of the energetics observed in herbs, foods, people, and illnesses, I'll list some resources for you to explore in the back of the book (see Appendix: Energetics of Common Ailments, page 179).

Pungent

The pungent taste (along with a close subset called "spicy") gets its activity from an abundance of resins and aromatic oils and is the hottest of all the tastes. Even in small amounts, the potent compounds in the pungent taste are stimulating, warming, and drying. The pungent taste brings warmth to the digestive system, which helps eliminate gas and bloating. These foods and herbs increase blood and lymphatic circulation, increase metabolism, stimulate immune response and sweating (promoting detoxification), and reduce and dry up excess mucus from the sinuses and lungs. Many of these herbs and foods also show antimicrobial, antiviral, and antifungal activity.

Some familiar pungent herbs and foods that have hot/drying activity: black pepper, cayenne pepper, chiles, cloves, garlic, ginger, horseradish, mustard, onions, and wasabi. In individuals with sensitive digestive systems, the pungent-tasting foods and herbs may aggravate gastric mucosa.

Spicy herbs are warming and stimulating, and constitute most of the common culinary herbs and spices that we use regularly. The spicy taste is carminative by nature and generally somewhat less stimulating, warming, and drying. Carminative herbs help increase appetite, promote proper digestion, and relieve gas and digestive cramping (after-dinner digestifs contain carminative herbs). They also stimulate function of the lungs and large intestine. Many are antiviral and/or antibacterial and have calming and antidepressant effects.

Some familiar spicy herbs and foods that have warm/drying activity: basil, bee balm, cardamom, cinnamon, cumin, fennel, lavender, lemon balm, mint, nutmeg, oregano, rosemary, sage, thyme, and turmeric.

Bitter

Not surprisingly, most Westerners choose to avoid this taste in favor of more appealing sweet or salty choices. Some might call the bitter taste an acquired one; however, it is well worth the initial effort. Bitter foods stimulate the liver, gallbladder, and pancreas to produce a multitude of digestive fluids and enzymes, and are best taken before meals. This prepares the digestive system for incoming food by properly breaking it down, which helps increase absorption of beneficial nutrients. As a bonus, bitter flavors stimulate peristalsis, thus improving elimination. These herbs are generally cooling and help reduce inflammation throughout the entire gastrointestinal tract.

Bitter herbs and foods have the most physiologically active flavor, meaning they stimulate more activity within the body than any other taste. Bitter herbs and foods can reduce cravings for sweets, stimulate metabolism and aid in weight loss, help metabolize fats and lower cholesterol, promote detoxification by cleansing and supporting the liver, and balance hormones. Many bitter greens are also mineral-rich; cooking them and adding just a splash of vinegar will help make these minerals more bioavailable.

The cooling nature of most bitter herbs and foods may deplete digestive fire if taken in larger quantities over a long period of time. It is recommended to combine the bitter taste with a warming spicy/pungent herb or spice to help balance and diminish this effect, for example, dandelion root tea with cinnamon, or kale with garlic.

Some familiar bitter herbs and foods include artichokes, arugula, collards, chamomile tea, coffee, dandelion greens, dandelion root, dark chocolate, endive, fenugreek, green tea, kale, orange and grapefruit peel, radicchio, and turmeric.

Sour

The sour taste is more prominent in foods, particularly fruits, than in herbs. Botanical compounds that contribute to the sour flavor are citric, malic, tannic, and ascorbic acids. Flavonoids, which contain a wealth of antioxidants, as well as vitamin C, are also present in fruits. Flavonoids strengthen and tonify the integrity of small capillaries, veins, and arteries. The sour taste is beneficial for the liver and the eyes, which both require more antioxidants than any other part of the body. The liver and gallbladder are also stimulated by the sour taste, which improves the appetite, helps metabolize fatty foods, and increases overall metabolism. Sour foods are used to cool and reduce tissue inflammation and tonify boggy mucus membranes in the sinuses, mouth, throat, and small and large intestines. The sour taste is cooling in small amounts but in large amounts over a period of time may cause hyperacidity in the digestive tract or aggravate acid reflux.

Some familiar sour herbs and foods include blackberries, blueberries, elderberries, grapefruit, hawthorn berries, hibiscus flowers, kefir, lemons, limes, naturally fermented foods (sauerkraut, kimchi, kombucha, miso), pickles, plums, pomegranates, raspberries, rhubarb, rose hips, sorrel, sour apples, sour cream, sourdough bread, strawberries, tangerines, tomatoes, vinegar, and plain, unsweetened yogurt.

Salty

Salty herbs and foods are nutritive, nourishing, and balancing. They provide the body with a broad range of beneficial minerals that restore and maintain electrolyte balance. Salty herbs regulate water flow in and out of the cells so they can send moisture to dry tissues while helping release excess moisture out of boggy tissues. Many of these herbs are mild, potassium-sparing diuretics that support kidney function. They also promote the thinning and flow of lymphatic fluid, so they soften swollen lymph nodes and thin mucus. Salt nourishes and strengthens bone, teeth, nails, and hair.

Some familiar salty herbs and foods include celery and celery seed, chard, chickweed, cilantro, dandelion leaf, lamb's-quarters, lovage, nettle leaf, parsley, seaweeds (like Alaria, dulse, kelp, nori, and wakame), and spinach. Seafood, such as oysters, clams, and anchovies,

DOSAGE

The recipes in this book focus on culinary amounts of herbs. These are amounts used to flavor a meal or make a single cup of tea. But don't underestimate their power. When used in cooking, the taste of an herb on your tongue (whether it is sour, pungent, salty, sweet, or bitter) will provoke different physiological responses in the body. By understanding and using these tastes to intentionally stimulate those responses, we can actively engage with our food choices for optimal health benefits.

At the same time, while a single meal or cup of tea may provide a physiological response that stimulates digestive processes or relaxes muscles, that activity will be limited in depth and duration.

To stimulate immune response at the onset of a cold, for example, consider adding elderberry to your diet multiple times per day in a tea or syrup. The same idea goes for sage or thyme in a poultry dish. As a seasoning, it would certainly add immediate digestive, antiviral, and antibacterial benefits; but drinking sage tea or oxymel (see page 160 for recipe) several times a day would have a more profound effect as a drying expectorant for a wet cough. These recipes will focus on the medicinal potential of the foods and herbs within them.

A note on pregnancy: Any herbal preparations beyond the gentle teas and culinary preparations in this book should be avoided during the first trimester unless working with a skilled herbalist along with your prenatal care provider.

are considered salty foods, as are naturally fermented tamari and miso, olives, hard cheeses, and smoked meats and fish.

The mineral-salt taste of herbs is unlikely to cause any adverse reactions. Those who have edema or high blood pressure should consume salty foods and condiments such as tamari, miso, anchovies, cheeses, and smoked meats and fish sparingly.

Sweet

In traditional Chinese medicine, sweet herbs and foods are contraindicated during acute viral conditions or when there is fever, respiratory congestion, poor digestion, diabetes, a feeling of exhaustion or heaviness, and parasites.

The sweet taste restores strength and vitality, and is particularly nourishing and rebuilding to immune function. The sweet taste, when used in moderation, is generally moistening and cooling. Sweet herbs are moistening to lung tissue in the case of chronic cold, dry lung conditions. Sweet herbs and foods are anti-inflammatory and healing to the gastric lining and the entire GI tract in the case of ulcers, gastritis, and irritation of small and large intestines. The sweet taste is also said to nourish and calm the nervous system. It helps us feel satiated and comforted. When used in excess (such as too many grains, fruits, or dairy), it can cause dampness, diminished digestion, increased mucus production, and sluggish energy.

Some familiar sweet herbs include astragalus, cardamom, cinnamon, fennel, goji berries, licorice root, and marshmallow root. In addition, many foods are considered sweet: bananas, beets, cane sugar, chocolate, cinnamon, coconut, cooked carrots, dark orange winter squash, dates, eggs, figs, grains, high-quality animal fats, high-quality meat and fish, high-quality milk and cream, honey, legumes, mangoes, maple syrup, melons, nut milks, nuts and seeds, prunes, sweet potatoes, tofu, and vanilla.

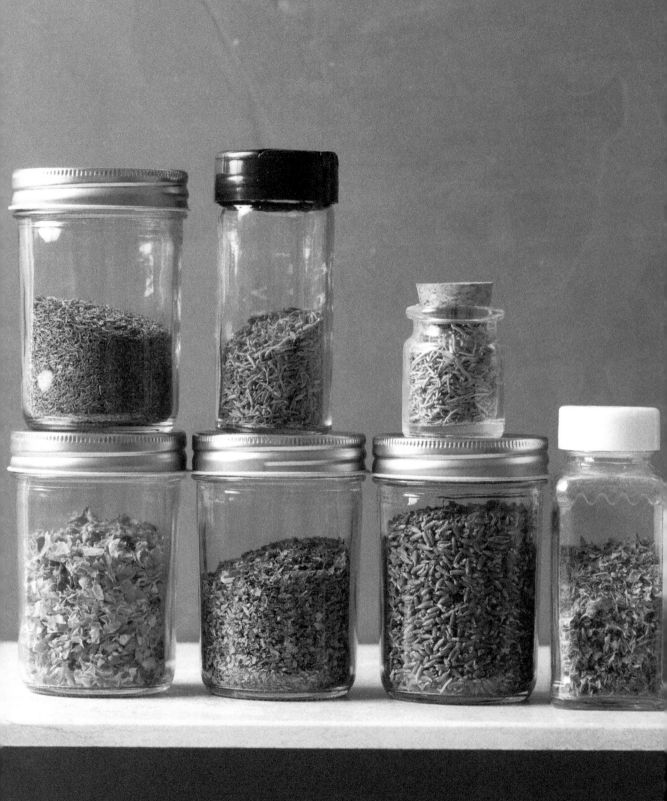

CHAPTER TWO

HOW TO COOK WITH HERBAL MEDICINE

If you enjoy preparing fresh foods from scratch or visiting farmers' markets to partake in abundant seasonal offerings, you're already halfway to understanding how to cook in a medicinal way. Do you like the piney, resinous taste of rosemary on garlic roast potatoes or sometimes crave a spicy meal during the winter months? Congratulations! You are intuitively on the path to stretching your taste buds and your senses from traditional cooking to medicinal cooking. Let me help you to fine-tune and expand the traditional knowledge that you are already using.

THE BASICS OF MEDICINAL COOKING

"Food as medicine" is a popular expression often used in the world of natural healing. But let's dissect that a bit. We spend a good portion of our lives eating food or thinking about eating food. If you are the chief cook in your family, you'll spend even more time considering budget and menus, shopping for food, and preparing it, too. Anything that takes up that much precious time in our lives should be embraced and enjoyed, shouldn't it?

In ancient China, the village physician was paid to keep its people healthy by teaching them how to use foods and herbal medicines while also advising on lifestyle and spiritual matters, if needed. Unlike our modern health-care model, if a patient fell ill in the village, the doctor was not compensated until the patient was well again. This holistic method of health care, then and now, shows the importance of maintaining balanced health *before* it declines. The easiest way we can do that is with the foods we eat every day.

What if you were given some basic tools to prepare simple, delicious, seasonal foods that automatically provided you with value-added nutrition and packed in some medicinal benefits, too? Taking the same amount of time to cook for yourself in a more conscious way is simply good "medicine" right from the start. With a little extra encouragement, you'll be enjoying food-as-medicine principles with ease at a cost far lower than buying monthly herbal supplements.

WHAT YOU NEED TO KNOW

You might be wondering how medicinal cooking differs from your current cooking methods. I like to use this simple analogy with my students to illustrate: Imagine you stop by the grocery store on your way home from work, planning to make a quick dinner. It is sleeting. You're bundled up, feeling a scratchy throat coming on. What would your food choices include? If your basket contained a cold prepared salad of chicken, lettuce, cucumbers, cheese, and eggs, and some watermelon, I couldn't say that these were unhealthy food choices. However, there might be more beneficial choices considering the season and your health needs on this particular day.

In my basket, I might gather chunks of winter squash, fresh ginger, garlic, cilantro, and curry powder to make a quick soup. At home, I'd slather elderberry jelly on whole-grain toast and make sage tea with honey. The difference between medicinal cooking and regular cooking rarely has to do with time or expense. It is simply understanding which food choices can gently bring your body back into healthy balance. Sometimes "food as medicine" is referred to as "tonic foods." This means that you can eat or drink them over a long period of time while they slowly and gently tonify your body. And rest assured, you don't have to worry about consuming a proper dosage or taking too much. Making educated choices about foods and herbs based on their taste and your own needs is fun and empowering. Let's get started!

SOURCING HERBS AND HERB QUALITY

Not all herbs are produced and processed equally. If you can grow basic culinary herbs in a backyard garden, in a community garden, or even on a patio, you'll have access to very good-quality herbs at a minimal cost.

The next best option would be to source fresh or dried herbs from a trusted friend or grower at an herb farm or farmers' market. Finally, you should always be able to find an abundance of fresh herbs at your local grocery store, year-round if necessary. Quality dried herbs are available online, or if you are really lucky, you might have a local herb shop within driving distance. I'll list some online herb sellers in the Resources section (page 185).

If you are reading this to understand the health benefits of herbs, you will probably appreciate the importance of purchasing from growers who don't use chemical agents on their plants. Certified-organic labels on fresh and dried herbs immediately show a trusted source for clean herbs. However, stringent standards are held in place by a governing body that requires frequent checks and documentation to earn its stamp of approval. All of this equates to higher-priced herbs, sadly. It's kind of discouraging to think that cancer-causing chemicals are cheaper than what it takes to keep herbs chemical-free. The good news is that many small, health-conscious farmers are growing chemical-free herbs without the added cost of USDA certification. Talk to your local gardeners and farmers!

WHAT YOU'LL NEED

You can easily adapt to medicinal cooking without a big change to your everyday kitchen equipment. I will list my most-used (and best-loved) kitchen tools right here:

- » Food processor for making quick jams, herb pastes, butters, and sauces
- » Slow cooker (4- to 7-quart capacity) for the convenience of making stocks and soups while you are away
- » Heavy-bottomed, stainless-steel soup/stock pot (3- to 4-quart capacity)
- » Sauté pans or skillets (8 inches and 12 inches)
- » Small saucepan
- » Ovenproof casserole dishes (from individual to family size)
- » Sharp chef's knife for chopping fruits, vegetables, and fresh herbs
- » Large cutting board
- » Wide-mouth mason jars (with some additional plastic lids) in quart and pint sizes for infusing vinegars, saving teas, storing leftovers, and making fermented foods
- » Wide-mouth funnel to fill your mason jars
- » Small fine-mesh strainer that fits atop the funnel
- » French press coffee pot (16 ounces) for making herbal teas with fresh and dried herbs
- » Stainless-steel microplane grater for garlic, ginger, citrus zest, and hard cheeses (so much easier than mincing by hand!)
- » Handheld stainless-steel skimmer/strainer for removing bones and vegetables from stocks
- » Stick or immersion blender for puréeing soups in seconds

Some personal preferences: I tend to avoid nonstick cookware, favoring my collection of well-seasoned cast-iron frying pans and enamel-coated cast-iron cookware instead. However, cast iron isn't for everyone as it heavy and does take some care.

BASIC HERB DRYING

If you grow culinary herbs, there is a quick and easy method to drying and thus preserving them. The secret to success is to accomplish it quickly away from light and humidity. Hanging bunches of herbs in your kitchen looks lovely, but it is not the best place to accomplish your goal.

» Wait until a bright sunny day to harvest and snip the top half to top third of the plant, stem by stem. It's said that the optimal time to harvest is before a plant goes into flower, but I like to include the flowers when I dry herbs. They are equally fragrant as the leaves and are a pretty addition to the jar.

» Remove any visible dirt, insect damage, or old, discolored leaves from your harvest. Avoid washing herbs unless they are very muddy or sandy. If you choose to wash, be sure to dry herb sprigs well between two towels before you start the drying process.

» Place a few loose sprigs into a paper bag. It's best not to crowd the bag as this will slow the drying process. Take your bag to a warm, dry location such as an attic, the top of a dryer, or even a hot car. Lay the bag on its side with the top partially open. This will allow for good air circulation and for moisture to escape.

» In a day or two, check your bagged herbs for crispiness, good color, and aroma. If you rub a pinch between your fingers and it crumbles, the herbs are fully dry and ready to store.

» Strip the dried leaves from their stems over a large bowl. Transfer the herbs to a mason jar, label, and store away from light. This will protect the vibrant color and fragrance from dissipating until your next growing season.

» To use, make tea (1 teaspoon for 1 cup boiling water) steeped 5 to 7 minutes. Or add to eggs, soups, stews, or sauces.

ABOUT THE RECIPES

This book is loaded with a wide range of recipes utilizing foods and herbs that are easily found in your own neighborhood grocery aisles. Some recipes may introduce you to new and different tastes, and others put a fresh spin on familiar favorites. I've made it my mission to use a minimal number of ingredients while offering lots of substitutions for different preferences. As a fan of three-ingredient basic recipes, I've included a few of these to encourage your own creativity, based on what is seasonally available or what your health needs are on any given day. Same basic recipe, taste-changed a few different ways! This helps avoid last-minute trips to the grocery store and inspires you to use up what's in your refrigerator or pantry.

FRESH VS. DRIED HERBS

If you are wondering if there is a difference between using fresh and dried herbs, the answer is yes! The main difference is simply intensity of flavor. When an herb is fresh, you'll need to use three times more than if the herb is dried. If herbal tea calls for 1 tablespoon fresh herbs for 8 ounces boiling water, you can substitute 1 teaspoon dried. Compare fresh peppermint to dried peppermint, and your nose and tongue will tell you that the dried is notably more concentrated. I prefer to use dried herbs in a tea or a long-simmering soup or sauce, when the hot liquids can release the oils that were concentrated in the drying process. I dry many of the herbs I grow so that I can continue enjoying them throughout the winter months.

However, sometimes it just comes down to texture. Fresh basil or basil pesto is vastly more fragrant and palatable than dried basil. The sticky, aromatic, pine-like resins of fresh rosemary leaves outshine dried leaves every single time.

I love to use fresh herbs in my classroom and kitchen during the months when they are green and vibrant in my gardens. I enjoy preserving that freshness in herb pastes and compound butters and freezing them for winter use. By creating herbal syrups, vinegars, jams, and spirits, I can capture the taste and vitality of seasonal herbs and appreciate their gifts all year long.

Within these pages, I offer a selection of recipes for breakfast, soups and salads, main dishes, snacks and sides, beverages, and a few desserts. In addition, a chapter on condiments features preparations for herb pastes, butters, vinegars, and syrups that can easily enhance—or even transform—basic dishes. These condiments are invaluable to have on hand in your pantry or freezer.

A note about pantry staples: I try to stock up a little bit every time I shop. If I discover a sale on organic canned beans (10 cans for $10, for instance), I take advantage of it even if beans aren't on my shopping list. Chickpeas mean hummus, white beans mean soup, and black beans mean chili or a satisfying Mexican meal. For $10, I have invested in 10 future meals. The same holds true for canned tomatoes, tortillas, vinegars, or coconut milk. Most of the recipes you'll find here can be made easily with pantry staples and fresh foods.

ABOUT THE HERBS

I've utilized the most familiar culinary herbs and spices in the creation of these recipes and explained how to use them in both their fresh and dried forms. In the condiment section, these value-added recipes describe how to best extract and preserve herbs so that they are at their most vital and potent year-round. In a sense, these condiments are your own personally created herb supplements. Making herbal condiments such as pesto redolent of garlic and basil or piquant vinegars sharp with infused sage or spiced elderberries will add another medicinal layer to your cooking without too much trouble at all. All of these various methods are provided to give you a wide variety of culinary and medicinal tastes, with the potential for great-flavored food combinations and, ideally, for sustained and improved health when used in daily cooking.

RECIPE FORMAT

Look out for the following items in each recipe:

Recipe labels: It's easy to see at a glance when a recipe is Dairy-Free, Gluten-Free, Grain-Free, Nut-Free, Vegetarian, or Vegan.

Yield: The majority of recipes are developed for four servings; beverages serve one or two.

Prep time/Cook time: As much as I enjoy cooking, I don't want to spend all day in the kitchen preparing a meal! Prep times are minimal and cook times are generally under an hour (unless it's a roasted meat or slow cooker recipe). There are just a few "Sunday afternoon" recipes that take a little longer to cook. Recipes labeled "Quick" can be made in 30 minutes or less.

Ingredient list: The recipes in this book are designed to use the smallest amount of ingredients packed with the most flavor. The ingredients are all easily found in your local food market except for one or two invaluable, key immune herbs, which can be easily accessed online. I'll list those for you in the Resources section (page 185).

Method: Everyone loves the idea being able to throw together quick, delicious creations. The recipes are designed to have a minimal number of steps to get you from pantry staples and fresh foods to a delicious meal in minutes. My goal is to follow a good recipe once or twice and then commit it to memory, so I don't have to read it a third time. I'd love to pass that simple pleasure on to you.

Tips: Each recipe offers helpful ideas on ingredient selection, substitutes, shortcuts, preparation, or serving suggestions.

Herb profile: A detailed overview of an herb or spice used in each recipe will list safety considerations, energetic properties, and medicinal benefits as well as a variety of suggested preparations and fun ways to use this herb in your medicinal kitchen.

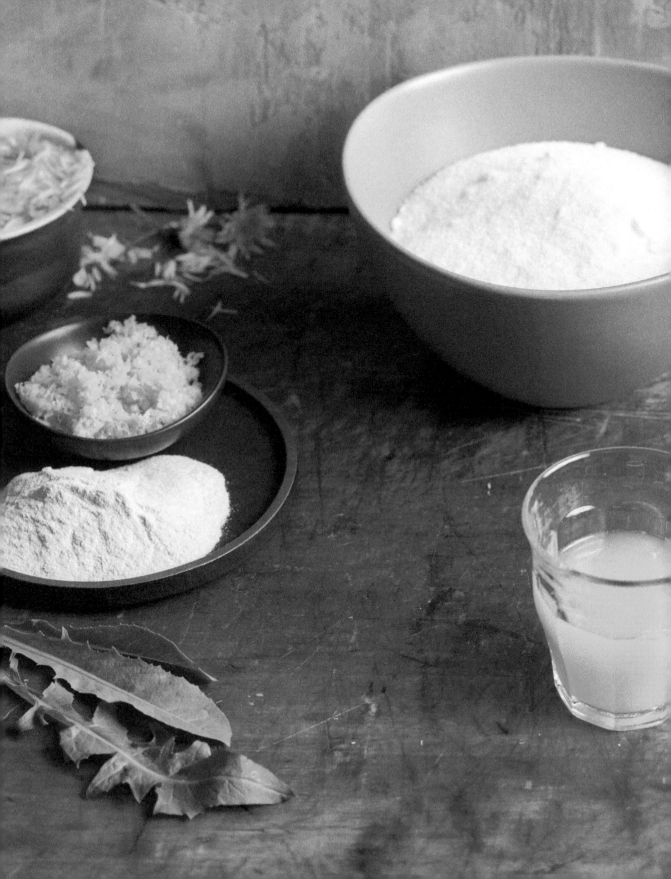

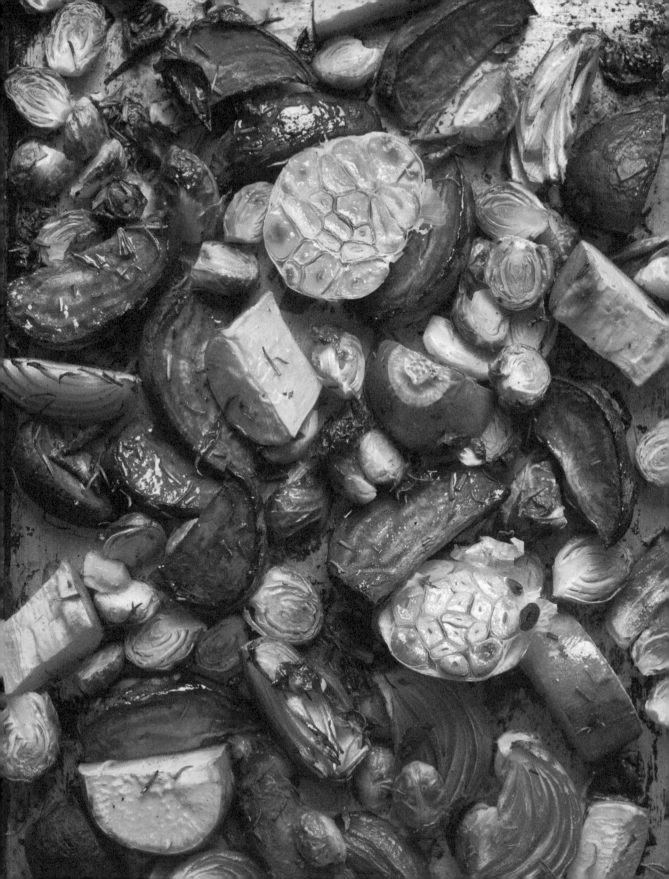

PART TWO

RECIPES

CHAPTER THREE

BREAKFASTS

When we "break fast" by eating bitter greens, healthy fats, pastured protein, and a good serving of fiber, it jump-starts the metabolism, gives us fuel for the morning tasks, and helps increase cognitive function so we can be more productive throughout the day. Add some organic dark roast coffee and you're in business.

I often think ahead to breakfast when I'm making dinner the night before, setting aside some steamed arugula or kale, salmon, or polenta. In the morning, it's so simple to add a fried egg and some whole-grain toast to complete the meal. Incorporating a healthy dose of pungent, spicy, or bitter herbs to the first meal of the day will also help increase metabolism, circulation, and digestion. And you'll get a nice dose of antioxidants to protect against the free radicals that age us.

Eggs with Polenta and Bitter Greens

This simple but delicious Italian classic is perfect for a hearty breakfast or an elegant light dinner. The bitter taste in foods helps activate the digestive process from the moment it hits your taste buds at the back of your tongue by increasing bile and digestive enzymes, and it may also help reduce sugar cravings and elevated blood sugar levels. The easiest way to incorporate the bitter flavor into your diet is to eat bitter greens on a regular basis. Here I've utilized my favorite, arugula, but see the herb profile for Bitter Greens (page 28) for a more extensive list.

GLUTEN-FREE, NUT-FREE, QUICK, VEGETARIAN

SERVES 4 | PREP TIME: 10 MINUTES | COOK TIME: 20 MINUTES

FOR THE POLENTA

½ teaspoon salt

2 cups water

1 cup polenta or corn grits

1 tablespoon unsalted butter

FOR THE BITTER GREENS

¼ cup water

1 to 2 tablespoons vinegar (preferably apple cider, balsamic, or wine vinegar)

5 ounces arugula (or substitute any other bitter green in the herb profile, page 28)

FOR THE POACHED EGGS

4 eggs

FOR THE BOWLS

Olive oil, for serving

Salt

Freshly ground black pepper

1 teaspoon lemon zest, for serving

Grated Pecorino Romano cheese and red pepper flakes, for garnish (optional)

TO MAKE THE POLENTA

1. In a pot, add the salt to the water and bring to a boil.
2. Add the polenta.
3. Stir well. Cover and reduce the heat to low, and simmer for 20 minutes, stirring occasionally to prevent clumping.
4. Turn off the heat, stir in the butter, and keep warm until ready to serve.

TO MAKE THE BITTER GREENS

1. Put the water and the vinegar in a medium-size saucepan with a lid.
2. Add the arugula and heat over medium heat. When the water begins to boil, stir once, cover, and allow to steam for 5 minutes. Drain and keep warm until ready to serve.

TO MAKE THE POACHED EGGS

1. In a small saucepan, heat 3 inches of water to boiling; reduce to a simmer.
2. One at a time, break the eggs into a small bowl and carefully lower them into the simmering water by slipping them from the bowl close to the surface.
3. Cook uncovered for 3 to 4 minutes. Using a slotted spoon, gently lift the eggs out of the boiling water.
4. Drain the eggs on a paper towel.

TO ASSEMBLE THE BOWLS

1. Place ½ cup warm polenta on the bottom of each bowl, followed by ¼ of the greens, and a poached egg on top.
2. Drizzle the top of each bowl with a little olive oil, salt, pepper, and a ¼ teaspoon lemon zest. Add the cheese and red pepper flakes, if desired.

COOKING TIP: If you aren't feeling confident in your poaching skills or need to make multiple eggs for a family breakfast, no worries. Simply melt 1 tablespoon of butter in a sauté pan and fry your eggs sunny-side up before topping the polenta and bitter greens.

BITTER GREENS

Arugula, collards, dandelion greens, kale, Swiss chard

SAFETY CONSIDERATIONS: None known

TASTE/ACTIVITY: BITTER/COOL/DRY

PROPERTIES: Nutritive

USES: Treats sluggish digestion and chronic constipation; aids absorption and elimination; stimulates liver, gallbladder, and pancreas

SUGGESTED PREPARATIONS: Raw in salads and juices is fine, but steamed or cooked with a splash of vinegar or citrus is easier to digest and increases the body's absorption of vitamins and minerals

ESPECIALLY GOOD FOR: DIGESTION

The bitter taste of greens can reduce cravings for sweet foods, stimulate metabolism and weight loss, help metabolize fats and lower cholesterol, detoxify the liver, balance hormones, and reduce inflammation. Many bitter greens are also mineral-rich. Cooking them will help make these minerals more bioavailable to the body.

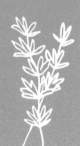

Breakfast Burrito with Spicy Sausage and Peppers

Give your mornings a powerful jump start with spicy breakfast sausage that includes digestion-stimulating spices like fennel, allspice, and cayenne. Adding a small amount of cayenne can have also have beneficial effects on the heart, blood vessels, capillaries, and blood pressure.

DAIRY-FREE, GLUTEN-FREE, NUT-FREE, QUICK

SERVES 4 | PREP TIME: 10 MINUTES | COOK TIME: 10 MINUTES

1 pound ground pork or turkey (preferably naturally raised)

1 small onion, minced

1 cup minced red bell pepper

⅛ to ¼ teaspoon cayenne pepper

⅛ to ¼ teaspoon red pepper flakes

½ teaspoon ground allspice

½ teaspoon whole fennel seeds

½ teaspoon sea salt

½ teaspoon freshly ground black pepper

2 tablespoons olive oil, divided

4 eggs, whisked

4 gluten-free soft tortillas

1 bunch fresh cilantro, washed well, dried, and coarsely chopped

1. Heat a 10-inch skillet over medium heat.
2. In a small bowl, combine the ground pork, onion, bell pepper, cayenne pepper, red pepper flakes, allspice, fennel seeds, salt, and pepper. Mix well without overworking.
3. Add 1 tablespoon of olive oil to the skillet and add the spiced meat. Use a wooden spoon to break up the meat while it cooks, allowing the meat to brown slightly.

〉〉〉〉〉〉

4. When browned, push the meat to one side of the pan. Add the remaining 1 tablespoon of oil to the pan and add the eggs.
5. With a spatula, quickly turn the eggs as they cook, combining them with the browned meat and vegetables.
6. Arrange the tortillas on a large cutting board and divide the meat/egg mixture between them. Sprinkle with a generous amount of cilantro.
7. Fold the bottom of each tortilla up and then follow with the sides, leaving the last side open.
8. If you aren't serving all 4 burritos at once, wrap them individually in parchment paper and refrigerate. They can be eaten cold or at room temperature within 3 days.

MAKE-AHEAD TIP: If you cook your spicy sausage and peppers on a Sunday afternoon, breakfast on the weekdays will be a snap!

CAYENNE PEPPER

Fresh peppers, dried peppers (whole or ground), red pepper flakes

SAFETY CONSIDERATIONS: May be contraindicated for people who suffer from heartburn, gastric reflux, or sensitive stomach

TASTE/ACTIVITY: PUNGENT/HOT/DRY

PROPERTIES: Anticancer, anti-inflammatory, antioxidant, diaphoretic, hypotensive

USES: Strengthens heart and circulatory system, treats diabetes, lowers cholesterol/triglycerides, aids weight loss, thins/loosens mucus in lungs and sinuses

SUGGESTED PREPARATIONS: Seasoning for eggs, meats, salsas, soups, and stews

ESPECIALLY GOOD FOR: HEART, BLOOD VESSELS, CIRCULATION

The compound that makes cayenne pepper (and all hot peppers) hot is capsaicin. Capsaicin stimulates circulation of blood in the body, strengthens the heart muscle and entire circulatory system, reduces blood pressure, and produces a phenomenon known as thermogenesis, a metabolic process that aids in weight loss.

Fresh Figs with Cinnamon-Spiced Almonds and Yogurt

This recipe provides a quick-to-make breakfast if you're on the go. If fresh figs aren't in season, substitute dried figs. The daily inclusion of cinnamon can improve peripheral circulation and lower blood sugar, cholesterol, and triglyceride levels in people who have diabetes.

GLUTEN-FREE, GRAIN-FREE, VEGETARIAN

MAKES 1 BREAKFAST BOWL AND 6 SERVINGS OF SPICED ALMONDS
PREP TIME: 5 MINUTES, PLUS 1 HOUR TO DRY AND COOL | COOK TIME: 20 MINUTES

FOR THE YOGURT

1 cup full-fat organic Greek yogurt

3 ripe figs, halved lengthwise

1 tablespoon maple syrup

⅓ cup Cinnamon-Spiced Almonds

FOR THE CINNAMON-SPICED ALMONDS

2 cups raw almonds

¼ cup pure maple syrup

1 tablespoon coconut oil

2 teaspoons vanilla extract

1 heaping tablespoon Ceylon cinnamon powder (see tip)

TO MAKE THE YOGURT

Put the yogurt in a bowl and top with the halved figs. Drizzle with the maple syrup and top with the cinnamon-spiced almonds.

TO MAKE THE CINNAMON-SPICED ALMONDS

1. Preheat the oven to 350°F.
2. Place the raw almonds on a baking sheet and toast in the oven for 12 minutes.
3. In a medium saucepan, combine the maple syrup, coconut oil, vanilla extract, and cinnamon.
4. Whisk until evenly blended and bring to a low boil over medium heat.
5. Turn the oven off and remove the almonds.
6. Using a wooden spoon, add the nuts to the hot syrup mixture. Stir to coat the nuts evenly.
7. Line the baking sheet with parchment paper and spread the coated almonds evenly on the baking sheet.

>>>>>>

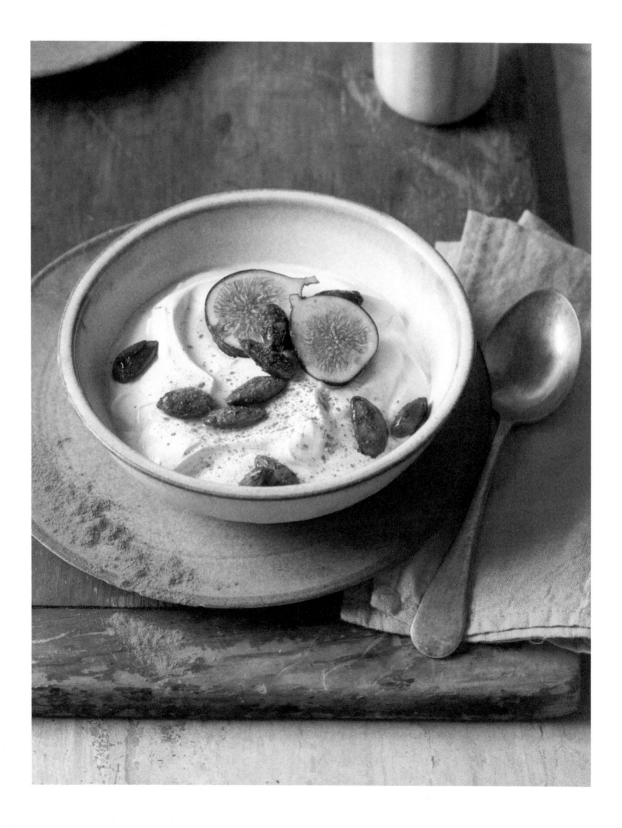

8. Put the baking sheet back into the warm oven and allow to dry and cool completely, about 1 hour.
9. Store in a sealed container.

MAKE-AHEAD TIP: Make your cinnamon-spiced almonds on the weekend or in the evening so they are ready to go in the morning or whenever you need a quick, spicy nibble.

INGREDIENT TIP: Both Ceylon (from Sri Lanka) and Cassia (from China) cinnamon are healthy and delicious. Cassia is the most commonly found cinnamon in U.S. grocery stores because it is very inexpensive. However, if you intend to consume daily therapeutic amounts of this spice (more than 1 tablespoon per day), it is important to note that Cassia has a high coumarin content. Large amounts of coumarin may interact with blood-thinning medications or cause liver problems. Ceylon cinnamon is considered much better quality, with only a trace amount of coumarin, but it is slightly more expensive. You can safely use up to 2½ teaspoons of Ceylon cinnamon per day. Look for clearly labeled Ceylon cinnamon in the grocery store.

CINNAMON

Powdered bark, sticks, chips

SAFETY CONSIDERATIONS: Avoid during pregnancy in more than culinary amounts. Avoid using with stomach ulcers and gastritis. Use cautiously with blood-thinning medications.

TASTE/ACTIVITY: PUNGENT/SWEET/WARM/DRY

PROPERTIES: Analgesic, antibacterial, anticoagulant, antioxidant, antiviral, astringent, carminative, circulatory stimulant

USES: Treats impaired circulation, cold hands and feet, chills, rheumatism, inability to sweat, cold damp conditions, intestinal viruses, diarrhea, poor digestion, foodborne illnesses (those caused by *Salmonella*, *E. coli*, and *H. pylori*), menstrual pain, cramping, scanty flow, fibroids, ovarian cysts, flu with muscle pain, diabetes, insulin resistance, and food cravings; stabilizes blood sugar levels; lowers LDL cholesterol and triglyceride levels; lowers blood pressure

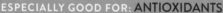

SUGGESTED PREPARATIONS: Baking, infused vinegar, syrups, tea, tincture

ESPECIALLY GOOD FOR: ANTIOXIDANTS

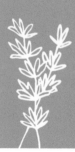

Ceylon cinnamon has the highest antioxidant content of all the spices, which may protect against free radicals. Free radicals can cause oxidative damage, which is associated with risk of arthritis, cancer, heart disease, and neurological diseases.

Dandelion Frittata with Goat Cheese

This delicious one-skillet meal goes from stovetop to oven to table in about half an hour. It makes a pretty presentation for Sunday brunch, too! Dandelion greens are loaded with minerals and vitamin C, which help build strong bones, hair, and nails. The bitter taste of dandelion stimulates digestion and absorption of those minerals. Combining bitter greens with eggs at breakfast is one of my very favorite ways to enjoy them.

GLUTEN-FREE, GRAIN-FREE, NUT-FREE, VEGETARIAN

SERVES 4 | PREP TIME: 5 MINUTES | COOK TIME: 30 MINUTES

8 eggs
½ cup milk
½ teaspoon salt
½ teaspoon freshly ground black pepper
1 tablespoon unsalted butter or olive oil

1 medium onion, minced
2 cups chopped dandelion leaves
1 medium tomato
4 ounces goat cheese, crumbled

1. Preheat the oven to 350°F.
2. Whisk together the eggs, milk, salt, and pepper in a bowl. Set aside.
3. Heat a 10-inch, oven-safe skillet over medium-low heat. Add the butter to the skillet.
4. Add the onion and cook slowly until translucent, about 5 minutes. Add the chopped dandelion leaves and cook an additional minute or two.
5. Cut the tomato in half, squeeze out (and discard) seeds and pulp, and chop into bite-size pieces.
6. Pour the egg mixture on top of the cooked onions and dandelion. Cook until the edges begin to pull away from sides of the pan, about 6 minutes.
7. Sprinkle the chopped tomato and goat cheese evenly across the top of the frittata and bake for about 15 minutes, or until the eggs are set.

8. Remove the frittata from the oven using mitts and allow to rest on the stove top for 5 minutes before cutting.
9. Cut into wedges and serve immediately. Leftovers make a great packed lunch either reheated or served cold.

INGREDIENT TIP: If you would like to add dandelion leaf to your daily health regimen, drinking it in tea form is another excellent way to extract those water-soluble minerals. Use 1 tea bag (or 1 teaspoon loose leaf) for 1 cup of hot water up to 3 or 4 times per day.

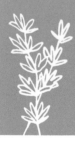

HERB PROFILE
DANDELION LEAF

Fresh leaf (for eating), dried leaf (for tea)

SAFETY CONSIDERATIONS: Do not use in the case of acute kidney disease

TASTE/ACTIVITY: BITTER/SALTY/COOL/NEUTRAL

PROPERTIES: Bitter tonic, digestive, diuretic, extremely nutritive, hypotensive

USES: Strengthens bones, nails, and hair; promotes liver health; lowers overall cholesterol/triglycerides; treats water retention and impaired circulation in lower legs; lowers blood pressure

SUGGESTED PREPARATIONS: Infused vinegar, raw or cooked, tea

ESPECIALLY GOOD FOR: BONES, HAIR, NAILS

Dandelion leaf is a super nutritious bitter green and an incredibly rich source of minerals and vitamins.

Slow Cooker Breakfast Rice Pudding with Chai Spices and Coconut Milk

The warming aromatic spice cardamom and lots of orange zest make this a digestive comfort food extraordinaire. Serve warm for breakfast or chilled for dessert. Cardamom has long been considered the elixir of longevity in traditional Chinese medicine. I can't think of a better way to encourage long life than to start the day with warm rice pudding. You will need a slow cooker for this recipe.

DAIRY-FREE, GLUTEN-FREE, VEGAN

SERVES 4 | PREP TIME: 15 MINUTES | COOK TIME: 3 TO 4 HOURS

1 to 2 tablespoons coconut oil

2 (13.6-ounce) cans full-fat coconut milk

1 cup water

1 cup organic white basmati rice

¼ teaspoon sea salt

1½ teaspoons ground cardamom

½ teaspoon ground ginger

3 tablespoons brown sugar

⅓ cup golden raisins

2 tablespoons finely grated orange zest, plus more for garnish

¼ cup chopped almonds, toasted

¼ cup chopped pistachio nuts, toasted

1. Coat the bottom of a slow cooker with the coconut oil.
2. Pour the coconut milk and water into the slow cooker, followed by the rice, salt, cardamom, ginger, brown sugar, golden raisins, and orange zest.
3. Stir gently to combine, and cover with the lid.
4. Turn the slow cooker to high. After 3 hours, check the consistency of the pudding. Stir well. If the mixture is too runny, cook for 30 minutes to 1 hour longer, or add more water if the pudding appears too thick.
5. Spoon into serving bowls and sprinkle with the toasted almonds, pistachios, and additional orange zest before serving.

MAKE-AHEAD TIP: If you have a timer on your slow cooker, you can assemble the rice pudding before bed, set it for 3½ hours, and wake up to a warm, fragrant breakfast. Otherwise, you can assemble your ingredients and turn on the slow cooker while you're making dinner, then turn it off at bedtime. It will be ready to reheat when you get up in the morning.

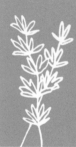

HERB PROFILE
CARDAMOM

Whole seeds, ground seeds

SAFETY CONSIDERATIONS: None known

TASTE/ACTIVITY: SPICY/WARM/DRY

PROPERTIES: Antibacterial, antifungal, carminative, expectorant

USES: Treats nausea, diarrhea, poor digestion of fats, gas, bloating, intestinal spasms, diarrhea, and constipation; inhibits bacteria, yeast, and fungi in the gut

SUGGESTED PREPARATIONS: Baking, chai tea

ESPECIALLY GOOD FOR: DIGESTIVE RELIEF

Carminative herbs and spices help reduce the formation of gas bubbles created by gut bacteria in the digestive process. Carminatives also help eliminate intestinal spasms, burping, bloating, and flatulence.

Gluten-Free Pumpkin Spice Pancakes

This hearty breakfast is the perfect start on a cold, frosty morning. Cinnamon in the pumpkin pie spice helps stimulate peripheral circulation, which warms up cold hands and feet, and helps lower blood sugar and triglyceride levels. The addition of pumpkin gives the pancakes a healthy dose of vitamin C, soluble fiber, and beta-carotene.

DAIRY-FREE, GLUTEN-FREE, QUICK, VEGAN

SERVES 4 | PREP TIME: 10 MINUTES | COOK TIME: 20 MINUTES

Coconut oil, for greasing,
   plus 1 tablespoon

1 cup gluten-free pancake mix
   (such as gluten-free Bisquick or
   organic gluten-free Bob's Red Mill)

2 tablespoons brown sugar

1 teaspoon pumpkin pie spice

1 teaspoon baking powder

½ teaspoon salt

1 cup coconut milk (or nut milk,
   if you prefer)

⅓ cup canned pumpkin purée

1 teaspoon vanilla extract

Maple syrup or nut butter, for serving

1. Generously grease a skillet with coconut oil and place over medium heat.
2. In a large bowl, stir together the pancake mix, brown sugar, pumpkin pie spice, baking powder, and salt.
3. In a separate bowl, combine the coconut milk, pumpkin, 1 tablespoon of coconut oil, and vanilla. Whisk until smooth.
4. Add the wet ingredients to the dry ingredients and whisk until just blended.
5. Use a ¼-cup measure to pour the batter onto the skillet for each pancake. Fill the skillet with multiple pancakes.

6. When the pancakes show air bubbles on the top, it's time to flip and cook until brown, about 1 minute.
7. Repeat with the remaining batter.
8. Serve with maple syrup or nut butter.

SERVING TIP: For a tasty, nonvegetarian treat, serve these pancakes with a side of maple-bacon butter: Finely chop 2 crispy bacon slices and put in a small mixing bowl; add ⅓ cup maple syrup and 8 tablespoons (1 stick) unsalted butter at room temperature. Blend well with a rubber spatula and transfer to a small serving bowl.

HERB PROFILE: See Cinnamon (page 35).

Avocado Toast with Heirloom Tomato and Basil Pesto

Avocado toast, while currently a trendy morning meal, will undoubtedly stand the test of time. It's a quick meal you can eat on the go. Avocado is loaded with monounsaturated fatty acids, which are good for heart health, lowering cholesterol, lowering systemic inflammation, and reducing the risk of cancer. In addition, the healthy fat in avocado fills you up and satisfies your hunger until lunch.

QUICK, VEGETARIAN

SERVES 2 | PREP TIME: 10 MINUTES

FOR THE AVOCADO TOAST

1 ripe avocado

Salt

Freshly ground black pepper

2 slices multigrain sourdough bread

2 slices large heirloom tomato

FOR THE PESTO

1 cup fresh basil leaves

2 or 3 garlic cloves

3 tablespoons walnuts

⅓ cup Parmesan cheese
(omit for vegan option)

⅓ cup olive oil

TO MAKE THE AVOCADO TOAST

1. Slice the avocado in half and remove the pit. Scoop the flesh out of the skin and into a bowl, and mash with a fork. Add salt and pepper to taste.
2. Toast the bread.
3. Spread the mashed avocado evenly over both slices of toast.
4. Top with a tomato slice and a big slather of pesto.

TO MAKE THE PESTO

1. Put the basil, garlic, walnuts, and cheese in a food processor or blender and turn the power on.
2. Add the olive oil in a slow stream from the top of the processor. Process until thick and pungent, which should take just a few seconds.
3. If there is pesto left over, spoon it into a small jar, topped with a thin layer of olive oil to keep it fresh and prevent discoloration. Cover with a lid and refrigerate.

MAKE-AHEAD TIP: Make the pesto ahead of time and keep it in the refrigerator for up to 2 weeks (if you don't eat it before then). Use it in everything from soup and pasta to eggs and toast!

SUBSTITUTION TIP: For a salty version, sliver 2 ounces of smoked salmon and press into the mashed avocado, along with 2 tablespoons thinly sliced celery. For a sour version, press ¼ cup mixed berries into the mashed avocado and drizzle with balsamic glaze (available in the grocery store next to balsamic vinegars).

HERB PROFILE

BASIL

Fresh or dried leaf

SAFETY CONSIDERATIONS: None known

TASTE/ACTIVITY: SPICY/WARM/NEUTRAL

PROPERTIES: Antibacterial, antioxidant, antiviral, carminative, cerebral stimulant

USES: Aids digestion; dispels gas and bloating; aids memory and concentration

SUGGESTED PREPARATIONS: Compound butter, infused vinegar, pesto, soups, stews, syrup, tomato-based sauces

ESPECIALLY GOOD FOR: ANTIOXIDANTS

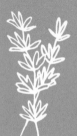

Basil is extremely high in flavonoids, a class of beneficial phytonutrients found in brightly colored fruits and vegetables. Flavonoids are powerful antioxidants that also show anti-inflammatory and immune system benefits. Diets rich in flavonoid-containing foods protect against oxidative damage associated with cancer, neurodegenerative diseases, and cardiovascular disease. Basil has potent volatile oils that also give it antibacterial and antiviral qualities.

Huevos Rancheros with Black Beans and Salsa Verde

Beans and eggs with a touch of heat is a classic cowboy breakfast. Here I've brightened it all up with fresh cilantro and a squeeze of lime. The fresh herbs and a salsa verde topping combined with eggs, black beans, and cumin give this dish plenty of fiber and antioxidants.

GLUTEN-FREE, NUT-FREE, QUICK, VEGETARIAN

SERVES 4 | PREP TIME: 5 MINUTES | COOK TIME: 20 MINUTES

2 tablespoons olive oil, divided

4 (6-inch) corn tortillas

1 cup prepared salsa verde (available in the grocery store in the Mexican food section)

1 (15-ounce) can black beans, drained and rinsed (see tip)

1 teaspoon ground cumin

4 eggs

Shredded Cheddar or Pepper Jack cheese, for garnish (optional)

Chopped fresh cilantro, for garnish (optional)

Lime wedges, for garnish (optional)

1. Add 1 tablespoon of olive oil to the skillet and warm up the tortillas, one at a time, over medium heat until slightly charred, 1 to 2 minutes per side. Transfer the warmed tortillas to a plate.

2. On each serving plate, place 1 warm tortilla, add ¼ cup salsa, and top with ¼ of the black beans. Sprinkle generously with the cumin.

3. Heat the skillet again over medium heat. Add the remaining 1 tablespoon of olive oil. Crack the eggs into the oiled skillet and fry until the whites are set but the yolk is still runny, about 2 minutes. Transfer 1 egg to each tortilla.

4. Add shredded cheese, chopped cilantro, or a squeeze of lime, if desired. Serve immediately.

SUBSTITUTION TIP: You can substitute a can of refried beans if you prefer.

CUMIN

Whole seeds, ground seeds

SAFETY CONSIDERATIONS: None known

TASTE/ACTIVITY: SPICY/WARM/DRY

PROPERTIES: Antibacterial, antioxidant, antiviral, carminative

USES: Stimulates appetite, improves digestion, and treats problems like diarrhea, colic, inflammation, bowel and muscle spasms, and gas; helps neutralize free radicals, which aids in cardiac health and age-related cognitive decline; may also help prevent diabetes and hypoglycemia

SUGGESTED PREPARATIONS: Black beans, flatbread, lentils, Mexican foods, refried beans, rice, tea

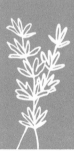

ESPECIALLY GOOD FOR: DIGESTIVE RELIEF

Cumin is a popular carminative in Indian, Mexican, and Middle Eastern cooking. Carminative herbs and spices help reduce the formation of gas bubbles created by gut bacteria in the digestive process. Carminatives also help eliminate intestinal spasms, burping, bloating, and flatulence.

Dandelion Marmalade

This is one of the easiest and most delightful ways to illustrate the concept of energetic tastes. Dandelion flowers (and their leaves and roots) have gentle but profound medicinal capabilities due in part to their bitter taste. Picking dandelions as a child is a pleasurable memory for most, and I highly recommend you "harvest" your own for this marmalade if you have time. An untreated lawn is the best place to find dandelion flowers in the early spring (avoid flowers by the road or ones that may have been sprayed with chemicals). It bears mentioning that every year Americans spend millions of dollars trying to eradicate this humble medicinal weed from their lawns. Embracing dandelion's nutritional and medicinal gifts instead could change the world in a radical way. You will need six (4-ounce) sterilized jam jars with lids for this recipe.

DAIRY-FREE, GLUTEN-FREE, GRAIN-FREE, NUT-FREE, QUICK, VEGAN

MAKES 6 (4-OUNCE) JARS | PREP TIME: 20 MINUTES | COOK TIME: 5 MINUTES

2½ cups sugar

¾ cup freshly squeezed orange juice

3 tablespoons grated organic orange zest

1½ cups yellow dandelion flower petals
    (most green bits removed)

¾ cup water

1 (1.75-ounce) packet Sure-Jell pectin

1. Place the sugar, orange juice, orange zest, and dandelion flower petals into a food processor bowl or blender.
2. Pulse together a few times until well blended.
3. In a small saucepan, whisk together the water and the pectin over medium heat until well blended.
4. Bring to a hard boil for 1 minute (no less). This step is imperative to create a thick marmalade.

5. Remove from the heat and immediately add the hot pectin to the sugar mixture while the processer or blender is running.
6. The marmalade sets up very fast. Have 4 sterilized jars and lids ready to fill, seal, and refrigerate.
7. Serve on toast for breakfast or as a glaze for chicken breasts.

SUBSTITUTION TIP: You can make rose petal jam using the same method above with these ingredients: 2½ cups sugar, ¾ cup water (instead of orange juice), 1½ cups unsprayed pink or red rose petals (instead of dandelion flowers), ¾ cup water, 1 teaspoon lemon juice, and 1 packet Sure-Jell pectin. Serve on toast for breakfast or use in Rose Lassi (page 158).

HERB PROFILE: See Dandelion Leaf (page 37).

Easy Fried Rice Breakfast Bowl

This hearty, Asian-inspired stir-fry makes excellent use of leftover rice or quinoa. The addition of salmon, mixed mushrooms, spinach, and scallions makes this an unconventional, but mouthwatering, breakfast bowl. The fresh grated ginger brings warmth to the digestive system and increases circulation to get you out the door with some warm, healthy fuel to burn until lunchtime.

DAIRY-FREE, GLUTEN-FREE, NUT-FREE, QUICK

SERVES 4 | PREP TIME: 10 MINUTES | COOK TIME: 15 MINUTES

1 tablespoon olive or coconut oil

1 cup mixed mushrooms (such as shiitake, oyster, and enoki), cleaned and coarsely chopped

1 bunch scallions (white and green parts), chopped

1 tablespoon grated fresh ginger, plus more for serving

5 ounces baby spinach

1 tablespoon water

2 cups cooked rice or quinoa

4 slices smoked salmon, slivered

1 teaspoon toasted sesame oil

1 teaspoon tamari or soy sauce

1. Heat a 10-inch skillet over medium heat and add the oil.
2. Add the chopped mushrooms, scallions, and ginger to the pan, and sauté until soft and fragrant, about 2 minutes.
3. Add the spinach to the skillet, along with the water. Cover until the spinach has wilted, about 2 minutes. Stir well.
4. Add the rice, salmon, sesame oil, and tamari. Stir to combine and heat through.
5. Divide into equal portions in four bowls. Add a little bit more freshly grated ginger on top, if desired.

MAKE-AHEAD TIP: This breakfast stir-fry is quick if you already have rice in the refrigerator, and sometimes it's worth cooking a little extra at dinnertime to make that happen.

GINGER

Fresh or ground dried rhizome (root)

SAFETY CONSIDERATIONS: Avoid in pregnancy in more than culinary amounts

TASTE/ACTIVITY: PUNGENT/HOT/DRY

PROPERTIES: Antibacterial, antiemetic, anti-inflammatory, aromatic carminative, circulatory stimulant, diaphoretic, emmenagogue, expectorant

USES: Relieves bloating, nausea, vomiting, burping, flatulence, low-grade diarrhea, motion sickness, and nausea from chemotherapy or antibiotics; treats cold hands and feet; thins mucus in lungs and sinuses

SUGGESTED PREPARATIONS: Baking, infused honey, infused oxymel, infused syrup, infused vinegar, tea

ESPECIALLY GOOD FOR: RELIEVING NAUSEA

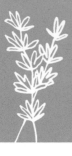

Ginger is best known for its beneficial effects for the digestive system. It can relieve nausea in pregnancy or caused by motion sickness, chemotherapy, or antibiotic use. Pregnant women with morning sickness should use only fresh ginger slices for tea. (Dried ginger is used as an emmenagogue to bring on menstruation; use is not advised during the first trimester.)

CHILLED GAZPACHO WITH LIME CREMA 52

PANZANELLA SALAD WITH TORN BASIL 55

BASIC CHICKEN BONE BROTH 56

ITALIAN WHITE BEAN AND ESCAROLE SOUP 58

SHIITAKE MISO SOUP 60

CURRIED PUMPKIN VEGETABLE SOUP 62

MEDITERRANEAN FISH STEW 64

RADISH AND ARUGULA SALAD
WITH MUSTARD VINAIGRETTE 66

CELERY SALAD WITH THAI PEANUT DRESSING 68

MEDITERRANEAN FARRO SALAD
WITH ASPARAGUS AND MINT 70

GREEK TZATZIKI CUCUMBER SALAD 74

FRENCH LENTIL SALAD WITH
ROASTED FENNEL AND ONIONS 76

CHAPTER FOUR

SOUPS AND SALADS

Soup is hands-down my favorite medicinal dish during the cold months of the year. I often start soups with homemade, collagen-rich bone broth simmered with immune-building herbs, and then bring in flavonoid- and carotenoid-laden vegetables, fiber-rich beans, and warming spices to keep inner digestive fires burning bright. This is medicinal cooking at its finest. I like to reserve cool, raw salads for the warmer months of the year, when garden vegetables and fresh herbs are at their peak availability and quality. The energetic foods, herbs, and spices in these recipes are specifically matched to the season so they can be prepared for optimal freshness and medicinal benefit.

CHILLED GAZPACHO WITH LIME CREMA

A recipe inspired by a dish my dear friend Hilda shared with me many summers ago, this soup evolves and changes every year depending on what is growing in the garden. When the forecast calls for triple-digit temperatures, mix this gazpacho together in the morning, and by dinnertime, you'll think it was the best decision you ever made. Because this soup is so quick and easy to make, I've included two cilantro-based toppings. The tomatoes and cilantro are both loaded with antioxidants that fight damage caused by free radicals.

GLUTEN-FREE, NUT-FREE, VEGETARIAN

SERVES 4 | PREP TIME: 20 MINUTES, PLUS 2 HOURS TO CHILL

FOR THE SOUP

2 cups corn kernels, cut from about 3 ears,
    or frozen

4 cups low-sodium organic tomato juice

2 medium tomatoes, chopped
    (about 2 cups)

½ English cucumber, peeled and cubed

2 ripe avocados, pitted, peeled, and cubed

½ red onion, finely chopped

¼ cup freshly squeezed lime juice

3 garlic cloves, minced

¼ teaspoon ground cayenne pepper
    (optional)

Sea salt

Freshly ground black pepper

FOR THE CILANTRO PESTO

2 cups finely chopped cilantro

2 tablespoons freshly squeezed lime juice

½ teaspoon minced garlic

¼ teaspoon salt

¼ to ½ cup olive oil

FOR THE LIME CREMA

4 ounces cultured sour cream or
    plain yogurt

2 cups finely chopped cilantro

2 tablespoons freshly squeezed lime juice

½ teaspoon grated lime zest

½ teaspoon minced garlic

¼ teaspoon salt

TO MAKE THE SOUP

In a large bowl, combine the corn, tomato juice, tomatoes, cucumber, avocados, red onion, lime juice, garlic, and cayenne pepper (if using). Season with salt and pepper. Cover the bowl with plastic wrap and chill for at least 2 hours (the soup gets better the longer it chills to blend its flavors). Stir the soup, ladle into bowls, and top with a generous dollop of the pesto and lime crema.

TO MAKE THE CILANTRO PESTO

In a small bowl, combine the cilantro, lime juice, garlic, salt, and olive oil and stir until blended.

TO MAKE THE LIME CREMA

In another small bowl, combine the sour cream, cilantro, lime juice, lime zest, garlic, and salt and stir until blended.

INGREDIENT TIP: Cilantro is usually grown in very sandy soil. The best way to remove the sandy grit caught within the leaves is to fill a medium-size bowl with water. Hold the bunch of cilantro by the stem ends and swish the leaves around in the water. You will see the sand sink to the bottom of the bowl. Change the water and repeat until the water is clear; dry well with a clean towel.

CILANTRO

Fresh or dried leaf; seeds are known as coriander

SAFETY CONSIDERATIONS: None known

TASTE/ACTIVITY: SPICY/COOL/DRY

PROPERTIES: Antioxidant, carminative, chelating agent

USES: Relieves gas, bloating, and nausea; relieves intestinal viruses, bad gut bacteria, and bacterial diarrhea; removes heavy metals in the body

SUGGESTED PREPARATIONS: Compound butter, fresh herb paste, in salads, tea

ESPECIALLY GOOD FOR: REMOVING HEAVY METALS

Recent studies have focused on cilantro's potential to remove heavy metals, particularly lead and mercury, from the tissues in the body. There has been both positive and inconclusive evidence to support this use. More studies are needed. Fresh cilantro is packed with antioxidants that prevent degenerative diseases like cancer, heart disease, diabetes, arthritis, macular degeneration, and Alzheimer's disease.

PANZANELLA SALAD WITH TORN BASIL

This is an exceptionally quick dish to assemble when your countertop is overflowing with ripe summertime tomatoes. Think of it as pizza in a salad! Both the tomatoes and basil are full of health-promoting antioxidants, and the anchovies add in a healthy dose of omega-3 fatty acids.

DAIRY-FREE, NUT-FREE

SERVES 4 | PREP TIME: 5 MINUTES, PLUS 30 MINUTES TO SOAK | COOK TIME: 10 MINUTES

4 ounces ciabatta bread, cut into 1-inch cubes

4 tablespoons olive oil, divided

4 or 5 ripe, mixed-color heirloom tomatoes (about 1½ pounds)

¼ cup red wine vinegar

3 garlic cloves, minced

½ teaspoon sea salt

1 red onion, coarsely chopped

2 ounces capers, drained

6 to 8 oil-packed anchovy fillets, drained and coarsely chopped (optional)

4 or 5 basil sprigs, stems removed, leaves torn

1. Preheat the oven to 350°F.
2. Toss the ciabatta with 2 tablespoons of olive oil. Spread the bread cubes on a baking sheet and toast in the oven for 10 minutes.
3. To make the dressing, cut the tomatoes in half. Scoop the pulp into a strainer set over a small bowl. Press the tomato pulp in the strainer to extract the juice. Then add the remaining 2 tablespoons of olive oil, vinegar, garlic, and sea salt to the tomato juice. Discard the pulp left in the strainer.
4. Chop the tomato halves into bite-size chunks.
5. In a serving bowl, layer the toasted bread, tomatoes, onion, capers, and anchovies, if using.
6. Pour the dressing over, toss, and let stand for about 30 minutes. This allows the bread to soak up some of the liquid and the flavors to meld.
7. When ready to serve, toss the ingredients once more, and stir in the basil leaves.

SERVING TIP: I like this recipe simple, with the best Italian bread, juicy tomatoes off the vine, torn basil, and fruity olive oil. But if you have no objection to dairy, a few creamy slabs of mozzarella cheese tastes wonderful in this dish.

HERB PROFILE: See Basil (page 43).

Basic Chicken Bone Broth

This value-added chicken broth not only forms a tasty foundation for soups and stews, but it also contains nutrients that build bones and improve joint health and amino acids that improve immune and lung health. A bit of astragalus root makes the immune-strengthening potential even greater. The apple cider vinegar extracts calcium from the chicken bones and makes your broth rich in minerals.

DAIRY-FREE, GLUTEN-FREE, GRAIN-FREE, NUT-FREE

MAKES 12 TO 16 CUPS | PREP TIME: 20 MINUTES, PLUS OVERNIGHT TO CHILL | COOK TIME: 5 HOURS

1 (3- to 4-pound) organic chicken

2 onions, coarsely chopped

2 carrots, coarsely chopped

3 celery stalks, coarsely chopped

16 cups cold water

2 ounces dried astragalus root slices (see Resources, page 185)

2 tablespoons apple cider vinegar

½ teaspoon sea salt

½ teaspoon freshly ground black pepper

1. Preheat the oven to 375°F.
2. Put the chicken in a roasting pan and roast for 1 hour and 30 minutes, until the skin is brown and crispy.
3. When the chicken is finished roasting and cooled enough to handle, remove the meat and set aside for another meal.
4. Put the bones, skin, pan drippings, onions, carrots, and celery in a stockpot and cover with the cold water. Add the astragalus root slices to the broth.
5. Bring to a low boil. Add the apple cider vinegar. Reduce the heat, cover, and simmer for 2 to 3 hours. The longer the broth simmers, the richer and more flavorful it will be. Remove from the heat and strain the broth through a colander into a large bowl or soup pot. Season the stock with salt and pepper.
6. When the broth has cooled, refrigerate overnight. The next day, the broth should be rich and gelatinous. The fat will have solidified on the top, so you can remove it, if desired.
7. At this point, your medicinal broth is ready to transform into a healing soup or tea or frozen in quart-size containers for later use.

SUBSTITUTION TIP: If you prefer a vegetarian broth, simply omit the chicken, double the vegetables, and roast them at 350°F for 40 minutes before covering with the water.

ASTRAGALUS

Dried root slices

SAFETY CONSIDERATIONS: Should not be used during acute respiratory illness with fever or with wet cough

TASTE/ACTIVITY: SWEET/WARM/MOIST

PROPERTIES: Adaptogen, antibacterial, anti-inflammatory, antioxidant, cardiotonic, hypotensive, immune amphoteric, mild diuretic, tonic

USES: Restores depleted immune health; treats cancer, chronic fatigue syndrome, weak or depleted lung conditions, dry cough, chronic bronchitis, high blood pressure, and diabetes; aids recovery from lingering illness or chemotherapy

SUGGESTED PREPARATIONS: Soup, stock, tea

ESPECIALLY GOOD FOR: IMMUNE HEALTH, LUNGS

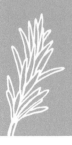

Astragalus is a tough woody root used in traditional Chinese medicine as a tonic to build and support the immune system. It is especially helpful for people who get sick at the beginning of cold and flu season and relapse or never quite fully recover, cough for weeks or months, or are subject to colds turning to bronchitis every winter. Use it to build up depleted immune function and lung health or to prevent colds and upper respiratory infections. Unlike the culinary herbs and spices featured in the book, astragalus is not used as a flavor enhancer. The woody root releases its powerful medicinal constituents when simmered for a few hours in water for tea or soup stock and is then discarded. Its taste is very mild and pleasant. Sip 1 to 3 cups per day beginning 6 weeks before cold and flu season.

Italian White Bean and Escarole Soup

This garlicky peasant soup is the go-to comfort food in our house when we feel a cold coming on or when the snow starts to fall. Don't let the small amount of ingredients or its short cook time fool you! This is one delicious (and medicinally potent) soup. The antibacterial and antiviral compounds in garlic help keep you warm and healthy during the cold and flu season.

DAIRY-FREE, GLUTEN-FREE, GRAIN-FREE, NUT-FREE, QUICK

SERVES 4 | PREP TIME: 10 MINUTES | COOK TIME: 15 MINUTES

6 cups Basic Chicken Bone Broth (page 56) or water, divided

2 (15-ounce) cans cannellini beans, drained and rinsed, divided

2 tablespoons olive oil

2 heads escarole, washed well and coarsely chopped

4 garlic cloves, minced

Sea salt

Freshly ground black pepper

¼ cup grated Pecorino Romano cheese (optional)

Pinch red pepper flakes (optional)

1. Using a stick blender or food processor, blend 1 cup of broth with 1 can of cannellini beans until smooth. Set aside.
2. In a stock pot, heat the olive oil over medium heat.
3. Add the chopped escarole, minced garlic, and salt and black pepper to taste and sauté for about 3 minutes, until the escarole wilts.
4. Add the remaining 5 cups of broth, the bean and broth purée, and the remaining 1 can of cannellini beans.
5. Bring to a boil, then lower the heat and simmer for 10 minutes.
6. Ladle the hot soup into individual bowls and garnish with the cheese and red pepper flakes, if desired.

HEALTH TIP: Did you know that chopping garlic cloves and allowing them to rest for 5 to 10 minutes causes the garlic to reveal its full protective, disease-fighting potential? Allicin, a beneficial compound in garlic, is responsible for its antiviral, antibacterial, and antifungal effects, and it increases as the chopped garlic oxidizes.

GARLIC

Cloves, dried powder

SAFETY CONSIDERATIONS: Garlic is generally considered safe but may interact with anticoagulant medications and increase the risk of postoperative bleeding. Some may experience heartburn or gastrointestinal irritation.

TASTE/ACTIVITY: PUNGENT/HOT/DRY

PROPERTIES: Anticoagulant, antifungal, antihypertensive, antimicrobial, antiseptic, antispasmodic, antiviral, carminative, circulatory stimulant, diaphoretic, emmenagogue, expectorant, immune stimulant, vasodilator

USES: Treats hypertension; lowers cholesterol; increases circulation; combats colds and flu, wet coughs, upper respiratory infections, pneumonia, bronchitis, sinus infections, and fungal conditions; aids digestion; brings on menstruation

SUGGESTED PREPARATIONS: Hummus, infused oxymel and vinegar (paired with other pungent herbs and spices, such as cayenne pepper, cinnamon, cloves, horseradish, and thyme), infused syrup, pesto

ESPECIALLY GOOD FOR: FIGHTING COUGHS, COLDS, FLU

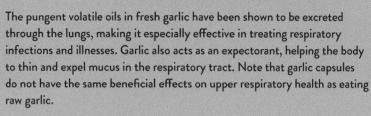

The pungent volatile oils in fresh garlic have been shown to be excreted through the lungs, making it especially effective in treating respiratory infections and illnesses. Garlic also acts as an expectorant, helping the body to thin and expel mucus in the respiratory tract. Note that garlic capsules do not have the same beneficial effects on upper respiratory health as eating raw garlic.

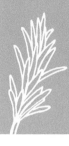

Shiitake Miso Soup

This soup is a clean and light, easy-to-sip offering when you feel like your digestion could use a little break, particularly after an intestinal virus or overeating during the holidays. The addition of miso paste provides plenty of beneficial bacteria to make you feel "right" again.

DAIRY-FREE, GLUTEN-FREE, NUT-FREE, VEGAN

SERVES 4 | PREP TIME: 10 MINUTES | COOK TIME: 25 MINUTES

2 tablespoons olive oil

1 cup shiitake mushrooms, stemmed and thinly sliced

½ cup thinly sliced leek or onion

3 garlic cloves, minced

1 tablespoon grated fresh ginger

2 quarts vegetable broth

1 cup thinly sliced carrots

1 cup thinly sliced baby bok choy

2 scallions, thinly sliced

4 ounces rice vermicelli

2 tablespoons light miso paste (available in the refrigerated section of the grocery store along with Asian or fermented products)

Soy sauce (optional)

Toasted sesame oil (optional)

Red pepper flakes (optional)

1. In a 3-quart soup pot, heat the olive oil over medium heat and sauté the shiitake mushrooms, leek, garlic, and ginger until the mushrooms are dark brown, about 5 minutes.
2. Add the broth, carrots, and baby bok choy, and simmer until tender, about 20 minutes.
3. Lower the heat, add the scallions and rice noodles, and cook for 5 more minutes.
4. Remove from the heat and let cool slightly.
5. In a small bowl, dilute the light miso paste with a small amount of warm broth and add to the soup (see tip).
6. Garnish with soy sauce, toasted sesame oil, and red pepper flakes to taste, if desired.

INGREDIENT TIP: A traditional ingredient in Asian diets, miso is made from naturally fermented soybeans and loaded with an abundance of beneficial bacteria. In Japan, people begin their day with a bowl of miso soup; it stimulates digestion and is often used for its regenerative properties after an illness. Because miso is technically "alive" with good bacteria, it's important to simply stir miso into warm soup at the end of cooking. Boiling miso will destroy its gut-healing properties. It lasts for many months (if not years) in your refrigerator. If gluten is a consideration for you, make sure to check the packaging for a gluten-free label.

SHIITAKE MUSHROOMS

Fresh or dried fruiting body

SAFETY CONSIDERATIONS: Do not use if you have mushroom allergies

TASTE/ACTIVITY: SALTY/NEUTRAL/NUTRITIVE

PROPERTIES: Adaptogen, alterative, anticancer, antiviral, blood purifier, hepatoprotective, immunomodulator, restorative

USES: Lowers cholesterol and triglyceride levels, restores depleted immune system, protects liver

SUGGESTED PREPARATIONS: Sautéed (not raw), tea

ESPECIALLY GOOD FOR: IMMUNE HEALTH

Shiitake is the most extensively studied mushroom. Shiitakes consumed three or four times per week can help lower cholesterol and triglyceride levels. They can also be used to reduce inflammation in the lungs, inhibit viruses, and prevent frequent colds, flu, and bronchitis. Shiitake mushrooms have been used in traditional Chinese medicine to protect the liver from environmental toxins, and research published by the *Journal of Clinical Oncology* suggests that eating shiitake mushrooms can help slow the development of some types of cancer cells.

Curried Pumpkin Vegetable Soup

Without a doubt, this recipe has been one of my most popular with family, friends, and students. It's made for a crowd, a few days of eating, or freezing. The beta-carotene in orange vegetables helps keep lung tissue healthy, so it's a good idea to keep this soup in regular rotation during the fall and winter months.

DAIRY-FREE, GLUTEN-FREE, GRAIN-FREE, NUT-FREE

SERVES 8 | PREP TIME: 20 MINUTES | COOK TIME: 20 MINUTES

2 tablespoons coconut oil

4 leeks, white parts only, chopped

4 garlic cloves, chopped

8 cups chicken or vegetable stock or water, plus more if needed

1 large sweet potato, peeled and cubed

1 (15-ounce) can pumpkin purée (or 1½ cups cooked fresh pumpkin)

1 (15-ounce) can diced tomatoes (salsa can be substituted here)

1 (15-ounce) can chickpeas, drained and rinsed

1 teaspoon sea salt

1 teaspoon freshly ground black pepper

1 (15-ounce) can coconut milk

2 tablespoons curry powder

1. In a 3-quart soup pot, melt the coconut oil over medium heat. Add the leeks and garlic, and sauté until the leeks are translucent.
2. Add the stock, sweet potato, pumpkin, tomatoes, and chickpeas. Stir to combine; add the salt and pepper. Simmer for about 15 minutes or until the sweet potato is tender.
3. Add the coconut milk and curry powder; stir well. If you prefer a creamier soup, use an immersion blender to purée the soup, adding additional stock or water to reach your desired consistency.
4. Keep on a low simmer until ready to serve.

SERVING TIP: For extra flavor, add any of these toppings to your soup: a handful of chopped cilantro, golden raisins, toasted pine nuts, leftover rice, frozen peas, or chopped greens, like arugula, spinach, or kale.

HEALTH TIP: To gain the best therapeutic benefits of turmeric (the main spice in curry powder), it must be consumed with a fat such as coconut milk, coconut oil, whole milk, ghee, butter, or avocado. Additionally, adding black pepper increases turmeric's absorption in the body by up to 2,000 percent. For best results, use ½ teaspoon to 1 tablespoon per day.

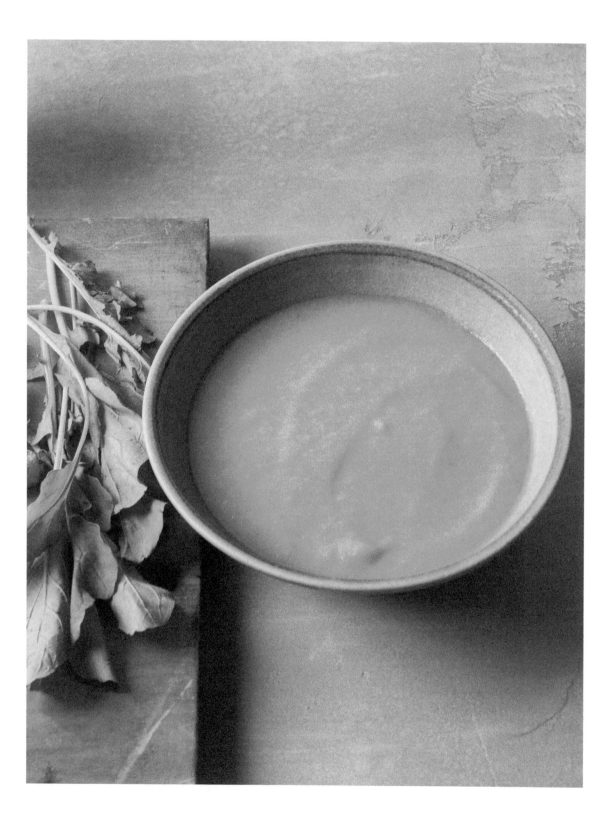

Mediterranean Fish Stew

This soup fills the house with the scent of bright citrus, wine, and fresh fish. An abundance of aromatic antiviral spices makes it a welcome addition to your winter cooking repertoire. Add some crusty bread with garlic dipping oil and you will be 10 steps ahead of any cold or flu in your neighborhood.

DAIRY-FREE, GLUTEN-FREE, GRAIN-FREE, NUT-FREE

SERVES 4 | PREP TIME: 15 MINUTES | COOK TIME: 35 MINUTES

2 tablespoons olive oil

1 cup chopped onion

1 green bell pepper, seeded and chopped

1 cup chopped celery

½ small fennel bulb, thinly sliced

2 teaspoons dried Hot & Spicy oregano

3 garlic cloves, minced

2 cups clam juice or broth

1 (28-ounce) can crushed Italian tomatoes or passata

1 cup dry white wine

1 pound wild-caught cod fillets, cut into 1-inch chunks

1 bunch fresh flat-leaf parsley, washed and coarsely chopped

Juice and zest of 1 lemon

1. In a soup pot, heat the olive oil over medium heat and then add the onion, pepper, celery, and fennel. Sauté for 5 minutes.
2. Add the oregano and garlic, and stir until aromatic.
3. Add the clam juice, crushed tomatoes, and wine. Cover and simmer for 15 minutes.
4. Add the cod, chopped parsley, and lemon juice and zest, and simmer for 15 minutes more.
5. Ladle into soup bowls and serve.

INGREDIENT TIP: Dried bee balm compares equally with the best Sicilian oregano (both are aromatic members of the mint family). If you grow bee balm, dry some in a paper bag and give it a try; it's not just for bees anymore!

OREGANO

Fresh or dried leaf

SAFETY CONSIDERATIONS: Avoid during pregnancy in more than culinary amounts

TASTE/ACTIVITY: SPICY/WARM/DRYING

PROPERTIES: Antibacterial, antifungal, antiviral, aromatic carminative, expectorant

USES: Treats colds, flu, wet coughs, intestinal viruses, sinus infections, upper respiratory infections, and fungal infections; aids digestion; relieves gas, bloating, diarrhea, and menstrual cramps

SUGGESTED PREPARATIONS: Cough syrup (with other warm/drying herbs for a wet cough), culinary spice, honey, steam inhalation, tea, vinegar

ESPECIALLY GOOD FOR: COLDS, FLU

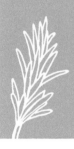

Oregano helps dry up excess mucus in the sinuses and lungs. Its antibacterial qualities may also help prevent any further bacterial infection associated with colds and flu. Oregano's carminative, drying, and antiviral activity may help alleviate symptoms from intestinal viruses, such as cramping and diarrhea.

Radish and Arugula Salad with Mustard Vinaigrette

I love the huge variety of multicolor radish seeds that are available and admit I probably buy too many packets every year! This salad captures the best of what my early spring harvests can offer. The bitter and pungent tastes stimulate digestion and activate metabolism after a cold, sluggish winter. This is truly a spring tonic salad.

DAIRY-FREE, GLUTEN-FREE, GRAIN-FREE, NUT-FREE, QUICK, VEGAN

SERVES 4 | PREP TIME: 15 MINUTES

1 bunch multicolored radishes

2 tablespoons chopped scallions

¼ cup olive oil

2 tablespoons rice wine vinegar

1 teaspoon maple syrup

1 teaspoon prepared Dijon mustard

1 tablespoon yellow mustard seeds

¼ teaspoon salt

¼ teaspoon freshly ground black pepper

5 ounces baby arugula

1. Wash the radishes and cut off the stems and roots.
2. Slice the radishes thinly using a mandoline or sharp paring knife.
3. Place the radish slices and scallions in a small mixing bowl. Set aside.
4. In a small jar, combine the olive oil, vinegar, maple syrup, Dijon mustard, mustard seeds, salt, and pepper.
5. Secure the jar with the lid and shake well. Pour over the radishes; stir to coat. Cover and chill until ready to serve.
6. When ready to serve, distribute the arugula among four bowls. Top each bowl with ¼ of the dressed radishes.

INGREDIENT TIP: There is a difference between yellow, brown, and black mustard seeds. The darker the color, the more pungent the taste. Yellow is by far the mildest tasting, but still adds some pungency to a dish. When you see a whole-grain prepared mustard on the grocery store shelf, you'll know that it will have more of a bite than plain yellow mustard.

MUSTARD

Whole seeds, powder, prepared whole-grain condiment, fresh greens

SAFETY CONSIDERATIONS: Avoid in pregnancy in more than culinary amounts. Mustard oils may cause digestive irritation in sensitive people.

TASTE/ACTIVITY: PUNGENT/HOT/DRY

PROPERTIES: Antibacterial, antiviral, carminative, expectorant

USES: Combats colds and flu, relieves congested lungs and sinuses, stimulates circulation and metabolism

SUGGESTED PREPARATIONS: Compound butter, infused vinegar, salad dressings (use sparingly due to its pungency)

ESPECIALLY GOOD FOR: LUNG HEALTH, RELIEVING CONGESTION

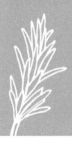

Most pungent spices (mustard included) have antibacterial and antiviral activity so are wonderful prevention for colds and flu. Mustard's sharpness also stimulates circulation and metabolism. In the case of congested lungs and sinuses, mustard provides relief by stimulating free flow of mucus.

Celery Salad with Thai Peanut Dressing

Oh, humble celery: always a supporting player, rarely the star. Celery is extremely high in potassium, calcium, and vitamin C. Here I've enhanced that age-old favorite combination of celery and peanut butter with classic Thai flavors. Adding some cooked chicken breast to this salad can supply additional lean protein.

DAIRY-FREE, GLUTEN-FREE, GRAIN-FREE, QUICK

SERVES 4 | PREP TIME: 15 MINUTES

1 bunch celery hearts with leaves, sliced at an angle (about 3 cups)

2 scallions, green and white parts, thinly sliced

½ cup grated carrots

½ cup chopped fresh cilantro

3 tablespoons smooth peanut butter

3 tablespoons rice vinegar

2 tablespoons freshly squeezed lime juice

2 teaspoons fish sauce (available in the Asian section of your grocery store)

1 teaspoon sugar

1 teaspoon sesame oil

2 garlic cloves, minced

½ teaspoon red pepper flakes

½ cup dry-roasted peanuts

1. In a serving bowl, toss together the celery, scallions, carrots, and cilantro.
2. In a small bowl, stir the peanut butter, rice vinegar, lime juice, fish sauce, sugar, sesame oil, garlic, and red pepper flakes until combined.
3. Toss the dressing with the chopped vegetables and chill until ready to serve.
4. Garnish with the peanuts before serving.

INGREDIENT TIP: It is important to note that celery is on the Environmental Working Group's list of the Dirty Dozen™, which means it is one of the most chemically sprayed vegetables around. Try to purchase organic celery whenever possible to get the most health benefits.

CELERY

Fresh stalks, seed

SAFETY CONSIDERATIONS: None known

TASTE/ACTIVITY: SALTY/COOL/MOIST

PROPERTIES: Antioxidant, diuretic

USES: Alleviates excess fluid retention; may help aid weight loss; helps to lower cholesterol; reduces blood pressure and inflammation; heals irritation, leaky gut, and ulcers

SUGGESTED PREPARATIONS: Celery seed tea (use 1 teaspoon dried seeds per 8 ounces boiling water), juice, raw, salads, soups, stews

ESPECIALLY GOOD FOR: ALLEVIATING WATER RETENTION

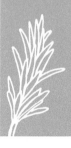

Diuretics stimulate the elimination of excess fluid in the body, particularly in the feet, ankles, and lower legs. Food and herbal diuretics help the body to expel water without depleting minerals, particularly potassium, which is a common side effect of prescription diuretics.

Mediterranean Farro Salad with Asparagus and Mint

My first introduction to eating vegetarian food came in 1980 at a summer potluck picnic where there were no fewer than six offerings of tabbouleh salad. It seemed so exotic to me at the time: cracked wheat, tomatoes, cucumber, and lots of olive oil, lemon, and mint. I was hooked. I've made variations of that dish every spring and summer since. In this recipe, I use an ancient grain called farro, which is loaded with healthy fiber and protein.

QUICK, VEGETARIAN

SERVES 4 | PREP TIME: 10 MINUTES | COOK TIME: 20 MINUTES

---

1 cup frozen peas

1 cup frozen edamame

1 (8-ounce) bunch asparagus, tough ends removed, cut at an angle into 2-inch pieces

1 cup uncooked pearled farro

¼ cup extra virgin olive oil

Juice and zest of 1 large lemon

1 handful fresh mint, cut into ribbons

Salt

Freshly ground black pepper

8 to 12 shaved slices Pecorino Romano cheese

¼ cup shelled pistachios

1. Fill a medium saucepan with water and bring to a low boil. Add the peas, edamame, and asparagus, and cook for 2 minutes.
2. Using a slotted spoon, remove the vegetables from the boiling water, and place in a serving bowl.
3. Add the farro to the boiling water and cook for 15 to 20 minutes. Drain well in a colander.
4. Place the warm farro in the bowl with the vegetables.
5. In a small bowl, mix the olive oil, lemon juice, zest, and mint together. Add the dressing to the salad and toss to combine.

〉〉〉〉〉〉

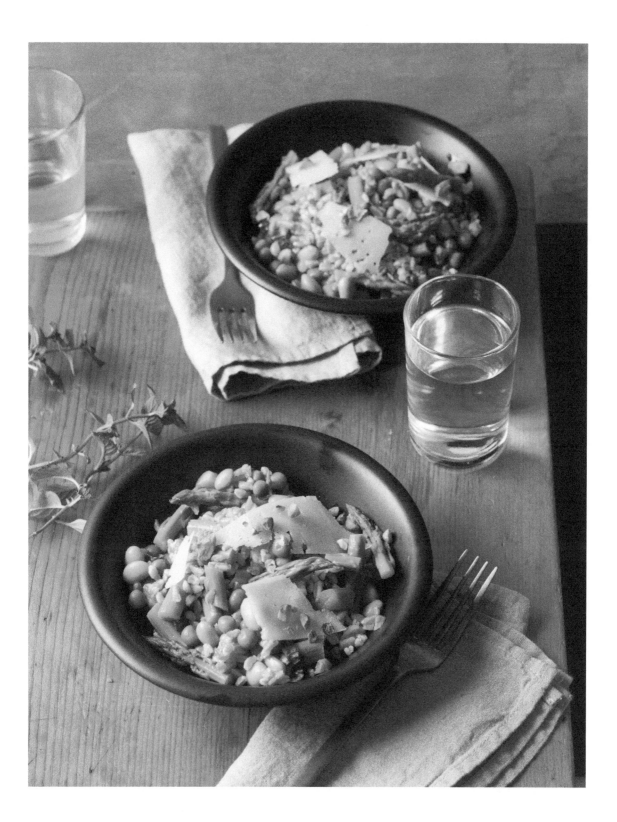

6. Season with salt and pepper, and garnish with the cheese and pistachios.
7. Serve warm or chilled.

INGREDIENT TIP: Farro is an ancient, minimally processed, and nutritious whole grain that contains 7 grams of protein per serving. That's more protein than either quinoa or brown rice. Although not gluten-free, farro has significantly less gluten than wheat. For those with sensitivities to gluten or concerns with it, this is important to note. This fiber-rich whole grain has a nice chewy texture and nutty taste. It is now easy to find in the rice section of most grocery stores.

MINT

Fresh or dried leaf

SAFETY CONSIDERATIONS: Some pungent mints, particularly peppermint, may aggravate acid reflux or heartburn in sensitive individuals

TASTE/ACTIVITY: SPICY/COOLING/DRY

PROPERTIES: Antimicrobial, antioxidant, antispasmodic, carminative, decongestant, diaphoretic (when taken as a hot tea)

USES: Aids digestion; relieves nausea, gas, intestinal spasms, bloating, morning sickness, and inflammatory bowel conditions (such as intestinal virus, colitis, irritable bowel syndrome, Crohn's disease, and diverticulitis); fights colds, flu, fever, and congestion; cools and relieves hot, itchy skin conditions, such as poison ivy and hives; awakens the mind and aids in concentration

SUGGESTED PREPARATIONS: Culinary herb, infused honey, infused syrup, tea

ESPECIALLY GOOD FOR: DIGESTIVE RELIEF

There are dozens of varieties of mint, and they may be used interchangeably. Some mints are less pungent in taste, such as spearmint and meadow mint. Others, like peppermint, have more potent and aromatic oils. My own preference is to use milder-tasting mints in cooking and stronger-tasting mints in teas, hot or iced. Carminative herbs and spices help reduce the formation of gas bubbles created by gut bacteria in the digestive process. Carminatives also help eliminate intestinal spasms, burping, bloating, and flatulence.

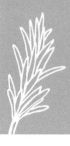

Greek Tzatziki Cucumber Salad

If you love the cooling taste of the Greek condiment tzatziki, you'll relish this full-fledged, full-flavored cucumber salad utilizing the same delicious ingredients. Dill is another prized digestive carminative that pairs wonderfully with cucumber.

GLUTEN-FREE, GRAIN-FREE, NUT-FREE, QUICK, VEGETARIAN

MAKES 2 CUPS | PREP TIME: 15 MINUTES

1 cup Greek yogurt

2 garlic cloves, minced

3 or 4 tablespoons chopped fresh dill

½ teaspoon sea salt

1 tablespoon freshly squeezed lemon juice

1 tablespoon grated lemon zest

1 English cucumber, peeled

1. In a small bowl, mix together the Greek yogurt, garlic, dill, salt, lemon juice, and zest.
2. Slice the cucumber thinly and place the slices in a serving bowl.
3. Pour the prepared tzatziki sauce over the cucumbers. Toss well to combine.
4. Cover and chill until ready to serve. Serve cold.

INGREDIENT TIP: English cucumbers are long, dark green cucumbers with very small seeds (or no seeds). You may substitute regular garden cucumbers in this dish. Just be sure to scrape out the big seeds (they can impart a bitter taste to your salad) by cutting the cucumbers in half lengthwise and running a spoon down the center.

DILL

Dried seeds, fresh leaf

SAFETY CONSIDERATIONS: Dill may lower blood sugar levels; caution is advised when using medications that also lower blood sugar

TASTE/ACTIVITY: SPICY/WARM/DRY

PROPERTIES: Antibacterial, antispasmodic, antiviral, carminative, digestive aid, galactagogue, relaxing nervine

USES: Aids digestion in the case of gas or bloating; relieves hiccups, diarrhea, baby colic, menstrual pain and cramps; treats diabetes

SUGGESTED PREPARATIONS: Culinary herb, warm tea

ESPECIALLY GOOD FOR: DIGESTIVE RELIEF

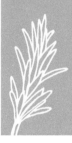

Dill seed acts on the digestive system to relieve cramping, spasms, and hiccups. Tea (1 teaspoon of dried seed per 8 ounces boiling water) also helps dispel gas and bloating. Dill and fennel together stimulate milk production in nursing mothers.

French Lentil Salad with Roasted Fennel and Onions

This hearty lentil salad entertains two different parts of the fennel plant: the fresh bulb and the dried, toasted seeds. The digestive benefits of fennel are well known for relieving gas, cramping, and bloating. The pairing of fennel and parsley along with the lentils is an especially winning combination.

DAIRY-FREE, GLUTEN-FREE, GRAIN-FREE, NUT-FREE, VEGAN

SERVES 4 | PREP TIME: 15 MINUTES | COOK TIME: 20 MINUTES

1 cup French green lentils

4 cups water

1 cup very thinly sliced fennel bulb

1 cup very thinly sliced red onion

⅓ cup olive oil, plus more for drizzling

Salt

Freshly ground black pepper

1 teaspoon fennel seeds

1 bunch Italian parsley, cleaned and chopped

¼ cup rice vinegar

Juice and zest of 1 lemon

1 generous tablespoon mustard

1. Preheat the oven to broil and position the oven rack on the middle setting.
2. In a medium pot, simmer the lentils in the water for 20 minutes while you prep the rest of the ingredients.
3. Arrange the sliced fennel and onion on a baking sheet, drizzle with a little olive oil, and add salt and pepper to taste.
4. Broil for 8 to 10 minutes, turning once, until fragrant and tender.
5. While the vegetables are roasting, toast the fennel seeds in a dry pan over medium heat until fragrant, 3 to 5 minutes (see tip).
6. Drain and rinse the lentils. In a serving bowl, toss the lentils with the warm roasted vegetables and chopped parsley.
7. In a jar, combine the remaining ⅓ cup olive oil, vinegar, lemon juice and zest, and mustard. Cover and shake to mix.
8. Pour the dressing over the salad, sprinkle with the toasted fennel seeds, and season again with salt and pepper.

PREPARATION TIP: Toasting whole spices is an age-old technique that releases and intensifies the aromatic flavors. It also makes your kitchen smell so amazing. Place whole spices in a heavyweight pan over medium heat. To prevent burning, keep the spices moving by stirring them with a wooden spoon or shaking and tossing the spices in the pan. Remove from the hot pan soon after the aromas hit your nose. Allow to cool in a heatproof dish.

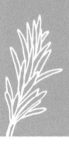

HERB PROFILE
FENNEL

Dried seeds, fresh bulb

SAFETY CONSIDERATIONS: Avoid during pregnancy in more than culinary amounts

TASTE/ACTIVITY: SPICY/SWEET/WARM/MOIST

PROPERTIES: Aromatic carminative, expectorant, galactagogue

USES: Relieves colic and teething pain in babies (when a breastfeeding mom drinks tea), gas, bloating, flatulence, nausea, and vomiting; treats intestinal viruses and dry cough; stimulates breast milk production; prevents mastitis; loosens congestion

SUGGESTED PREPARATIONS: After-dinner digestif, culinary spice, fresh bulb roasted and sliced in salad, tea

ESPECIALLY GOOD FOR: DIGESTIVE RELIEF

Fennel relieves gas, vomiting, nausea, burping, flatulence, and chronic low-grade diarrhea.

SUNDAY ROAST CHICKEN
WITH CHIMICHURRI SAUCE 80

POOR MAN'S "CRAB" CAKES
WITH YOGURT DILL SAUCE 83

PORK LOIN WITH ELDERBERRY PLUM CHUTNEY 85

ELDERBERRY PLUM CHUTNEY 86

PENNSYLVANIA DUTCH CORN PIE
WITH DANDELION GREENS 88

OVEN-ROASTED CHICKEN SATAY 89

NONNA'S ITALIAN MEATBALLS 90

SUMMER RATATOUILLE WITH CHICKPEAS 92

CLASSIC BEEF STEW 95

STIR-FRY WITH CHICKEN AND 3 CABBAGES 98

PASTA WITH PROSCIUTTO AND PEAS 99

CHILI COD TACOS WITH LIME CREMA 100

SPANISH RICE ZUCCHINI BOATS 103

QUICK PAD THAI 104

"THE GREEK" LAMB BURGER WITH
FETA CHEESE AND TZATZIKI 106

CHAPTER FIVE

MAIN DISHES

The main meal honors the gathering of hungry souls back home at the end of the day. In this chapter, there are quick weeknight recipes and those that celebrate the beauty of a slow-cooked weekend repast. I'll shine a light on the pungent, warming, and immune-stimulating qualities of garlic, oregano, chiles, cumin, ginger, and even elderberries.

I am a firm believer in the healing power of recipes passed down through familial generations and a meal prepared with love, laughter, and good memories infused into it. Since these are equally important to good health and a sturdy immune system, I urge you to cook with others, share a meal, or plan a potluck as you establish your own medicinal kitchen.

Sunday Roast Chicken with Chimichurri Sauce

I love roasting a chicken on Sundays. You can easily make use of the leftover bones, neck, and giblets by making mineral-rich, immune-building stock (see Basic Chicken Bone Broth, page 56). This moist, flavorful chicken can easily stand on its own, but when I have lots of extra parsley, I am inspired to make an Argentinian favorite: chimichurri sauce. It's totally green, uses plenty of parsley, and is loaded with antioxidants, vitamin C, and a bit of heat from chile pepper. This flavorful sauce whips up in mere seconds while the chicken is roasting, and any leftovers can be served with eggs or rice the next day.

DAIRY-FREE, GLUTEN-FREE, GRAIN-FREE, NUT-FREE

SERVES 4 | PREP TIME: 20 MINUTES | COOK TIME: 1 HOUR 30 MINUTES

FOR THE ROAST CHICKEN

1 (3- to 4-pound) whole chicken

2 tablespoons olive oil

½ teaspoon salt

½ teaspoon freshly ground black pepper

4 garlic cloves

1 lemon

FOR THE CHIMICHURRI SAUCE

1 cup finely chopped fresh parsley leaves

3 garlic cloves, minced

½ cup olive oil

3 tablespoons red wine vinegar

1 small red chile, seeded and minced
  (or 1 teaspoon red pepper flakes)

¾ teaspoon dried oregano

1 teaspoon coarse salt

½ teaspoon freshly ground black pepper

1. Preheat the oven to 400°F.
2. Remove the giblets and neck from the chicken, discard any packaging, and place them in the roasting pan. Even if you don't plan on eating them, these add good flavor to stock.
3. Rinse out the inside of the chicken under cool running water, pat dry with a paper towel, and place in the roasting pan.
4. Rub the entire chicken with the olive oil, then sprinkle it generously inside and out with the salt and pepper.
5. Smash the garlic cloves with the flat side of your knife and cut the lemon in half. Stuff it all into the cavity of the chicken.
6. Add an inch or two of water to the bottom of the roasting pan. This will ensure a moist chicken and allow you to baste with the pan juices every half hour, if desired.
7. Place the chicken in the oven and roast for 1½ hours. The skin should be brown and crispy, and the juices should run clear. The wings and legs should be loose if wiggled. If you have a meat thermometer, stick it into the meatiest part of the breast; the temperature should register 180°F.
8. Let the chicken rest for at least 10 minutes before you carve it to allow the juices to sink back into the meat.

TO MAKE THE CHIMICHURRI SAUCE

While the chicken is roasting, mix the parsley, garlic, olive oil, vinegar, chile, oregano, salt, and pepper together thoroughly in a bowl. Baste the chicken with the sauce and/or use as a garnish when serving. (If the sauce comes into contact with raw or partially cooked chicken, discard any leftovers.)

SUBSTITUTION TIP: Chimichurri is all about the parsley, but you can split the parsley in the recipe 50/50 with cilantro for more bite.

HERB PROFILE: See Garlic (page 59).

PARSLEY

Fresh or dried leaf

SAFETY CONSIDERATIONS: Avoid during pregnancy in more than culinary amounts (dries up breast milk)

TASTE/ACTIVITY: SALT/WARM/DRY

PROPERTIES: Antioxidant, carminative, nutritive

USES: Treats edema and poor fluid circulation in legs; stimulates kidney function; provides nutrition

SUGGESTED PREPARATIONS: Culinary herb, fresh in condiments, juice, tea

ESPECIALLY GOOD FOR: NUTRITION

Nutritive herbs are vitamin- and mineral-rich food sources. Parsley can be used as a food daily, if desired. It is extremely high in vitamin C. Drinking teas and vinegars infused with nutritive herbs is the best way to extract minerals such as calcium, magnesium, potassium, silica, zinc, and iron.

Poor Man's "Crab" Cakes with Yogurt Dill Sauce

These crispy, panfried, shellfish-free summer squash cakes are a delicious way to celebrate the abundance of zucchini and yellow summer squash. Cocktail and tartar sauces are the standard fit for crab cakes, but I've created a fresh, piquant yogurt dill sauce to elevate the lowly squash cake to rich standards! Add a toasted English muffin on the bottom and a poached or panfried egg on top, slather in sauce, and you have a lovely light brunch, lunch, or dinner.

NUT-FREE, QUICK, VEGETARIAN

SERVES 6 | PREP TIME: 10 MINUTES | COOK TIME: 10 MINUTES

FOR THE "CRAB" CAKES

- 1 cup bread crumbs (not gluten-free), plus more if needed
- 2 cups grated zucchini and/or yellow squash (about 3 medium), moisture pressed out firmly with a clean linen towel
- 3 tablespoons Greek yogurt
- 1 egg, beaten
- 2 to 3 teaspoons Old Bay seasoning (or to taste)
- 1 tablespoon minced fresh parsley
- ¼ teaspoon freshly ground black pepper
- 1 small onion, finely chopped
- 2 tablespoons olive oil

FOR YOGURT DILL SAUCE

- ½ cup Greek yogurt
- 1 tablespoon freshly squeezed lemon juice
- 1 tablespoon capers, drained
- 1 tablespoon finely chopped fresh dill
- 1 garlic clove, minced

〉〉〉〉〉〉

Poor Man's "Crab" Cakes with Yogurt Dill Sauce (continued)

TO MAKE THE "CRAB" CAKES

1. Pour the bread crumbs into a medium bowl. Add the squash, yogurt, egg, Old Bay seasoning, parsley, pepper, and onion. Let the mixture rest for a few minutes.
2. The mixture should be firm and hold together well, and not be too wet. Add more bread crumbs if necessary and form into 6 patties.
3. Heat the olive oil in a skillet over medium heat. Add the squash cakes to the pan.
4. Cook until nicely golden, about 5 minutes per side.

TO MAKE THE YOGURT DILL SAUCE

Combine the yogurt, lemon juice, capers, dill, and garlic in a small bowl and stir until well mixed. Serve as an accompaniment to the squash cakes.

INGREDIENT TIP: I love to use gluten-free bread crumbs wherever possible, but unfortunately, in this recipe they result in gooey squash cakes. The moisture from the shredded zucchini combined with rice starch bread crumbs don't allow the cakes to firm up as well as the traditional version.

HERB PROFILE: See Dill (page 75).

Pork Loin with Elderberry Plum Chutney

Loaded with vitamin C, antioxidants, and warming spices, the elderberry plum chutney is the star of this dish. Elderberries pack an antiviral punch when used for cold and flu prevention. Used as a delicious glaze on the pork loin in this recipe, it also makes a spicy condiment for wraps or a winning side dish with curries. I would even encourage you to try it straight from the spoon up to four times a day at the first sign of a cold. It is certainly a winter favorite in our house.

DAIRY-FREE, GLUTEN-FREE, GRAIN-FREE, NUT-FREE

SERVES 4 | PREP TIME: 15 MINUTES, PLUS 10 MINUTES TO REST | COOK TIME: 20 MINUTES

1½ pounds boneless pork tenderloin

2 tablespoons olive oil, divided

½ teaspoon salt

½ teaspoon coarsely ground black pepper

½ teaspoon garlic powder

Elderberry Plum Chutney (page 86), for basting and serving

1. Preheat the oven to 400°F and place the rack on the middle setting.
2. Trim the tenderloin of any fat or silver skin, and pat dry with a paper towel. Pierce the pork loin all over with a fork and rub with 1 tablespoon of olive oil.
3. Season the pork loin generously with the salt, coarse black pepper, and garlic powder.
4. Heat the remaining 1 tablespoon of olive oil in a large ovenproof skillet over medium-high heat.
5. Once the oil is hot, add the pork and brown on all sides, about 5 minutes total. Remove from the heat.
6. Spoon ¼ cup of the chutney over the meat, coating as much as possible.
7. Place the skillet in the oven and roast, uncovered, for 15 minutes, flipping the tenderloin over halfway through, until the center of the pork registers at least 150°F on a meat thermometer.
8. Transfer the meat to a cutting board, cover with a length of aluminum foil, and let rest for 5 to 10 minutes.
9. Slice the pork into ½-inch-thick rounds and serve with additional chutney.

ELDERBERRY PLUM CHUTNEY

Loaded with vitamin C, antioxidants, and warming spices, the elderberry plum chutney is the star of this dish. Elderberries pack an antiviral punch when used for cold and flu prevention. Used as a delicious glaze on the pork loin in this recipe, it also makes a spicy condiment for wraps or a winning side dish with curries. I would even encourage you to try it straight from the spoon up to four times a day at the first sign of a cold. It is certainly a winter favorite in our house.

DAIRY-FREE, GLUTEN-FREE, GRAIN-FREE, NUT-FREE

MAKES 1 PINT | PREP TIME: 15 MINUTES | COOK TIME: 45 MINUTES

½ cup red onion, chopped

1 tablespoon olive oil

4 dark plums, pitted and chopped (about 2 cups)

½ cup dried rose hips (or raisins)

¾ cup sugar

1 teaspoon ground cinnamon

½ teaspoon ground ginger

½ teaspoon dried cloves

1 cup Elderberry Vinegar (page 130)

1. In a 2-quart saucepan, sauté the onion in the olive oil over medium heat, stirring constantly until translucent, about 5 minutes.
2. Add the plums, rose hips, sugar, cinnamon, ginger, cloves, and elderberry vinegar. Reduce the heat to medium-low and cook, uncovered, until the fruit has collapsed and the mixture has thickened, about 25 minutes. Stir often to prevent sticking.
3. Allow the chutney to cool, and spoon into a pint-size mason jar. Store in the refrigerator for up to 6 months (if you don't devour it first!)

HEALTH TIP: Dark red, blue, and purple-pigmented foods are naturally high in beneficial antioxidants called anthocyanins, which are beneficial for cardiovascular health, cancer prevention, and regulating glucose levels. Elderberries specifically are at the top of my list for cold and flu prevention due to their high levels of antiviral activity. Elderberry preparations, such as teas, syrups, vinegars, shrubs, and jellies, can promote respiratory health, soothe upper respiratory inflammation, and act as an expectorant for congested lungs.

ELDERBERRY

Fresh cooked (not raw) or dried berries

SAFETY CONSIDERATIONS: Fresh elderberries cannot be eaten raw or juiced. The seeds contain cyanide compounds that would cause digestive distress if consumed. When berries are cooked or dried, the cyanide dissipates, making them safe to eat.

TASTE/ACTIVITY: SOUR/SWEET/COOL/DRY

PROPERTIES: Anti-inflammatory, antioxidant, antiviral, decongestant, mild laxative

USES: Prevents colds and flu, relieves congestion

SUGGESTED PREPARATIONS: Infused oxymel, infused syrup, infused vinegar, tea

ESPECIALLY GOOD FOR: COLD AND FLU PREVENTION

Elderberry products are well known for their antiviral properties. They are helpful for warding off colds and flu prophylactically and at the first sign of symptoms. The berries contain vitamin C and flavonoids, which can reduce allergy symptoms, congestion, and irritation in the sinuses.

Pennsylvania Dutch Corn Pie with Dandelion Greens

When making this family-favorite recipe over the years, I've stirred in hefty helpings of dandelion greens and parsley to add extra vitamin C and bone-building minerals. To save time in the kitchen, I've made this recipe crust-free.

GLUTEN-FREE, NUT-FREE

SERVES 4 TO 6 | PREP TIME: 20 MINUTES | COOK TIME: 45 MINUTES

6 eggs

1½ cups half and half

4 slices bacon

2 cups corn kernels, cut from about 3 ears or frozen

3 scallions, thinly sliced

½ cup chopped dandelion greens

½ cup chopped parsley

Dash salt

Dash freshly ground black pepper

Butter, for greasing

1 cup gluten-free panko bread crumbs

1 tablespoon olive oil

1. Preheat the oven to 400°F.
2. In a medium bowl, beat the eggs and add the half and half. Set aside.
3. Cook the bacon, drain, and chop into bite-size pieces. Set aside.
4. Combine the egg mixture with the corn, bacon, scallions, dandelion greens, parsley, salt, and pepper.
5. Generously grease a 10-inch pie plate with the butter, then pour in the egg mixture.
6. Toss the bread crumbs with the olive oil in a small bowl, then distribute them across the top.
7. Bake for 40 to 45 minutes, or until the eggs are set. Serve warm.

SERVING TIP: This pie will serve up like a crustless quiche. A side of cucumber salad or freshly sliced tomatoes turns this into the ultimate summertime meal.

HERB PROFILE: See Dandelion Leaf (page 37) and Parsley (page 82).

Oven-Roasted Chicken Satay

Chicken satay is a family favorite we've always enjoyed at our local Thai restaurant. But when I moved 100 miles away from that wonderful place, I had to learn to make it myself. To shorten prep time, I omit the skewers and grilling. Instead, I add all of the spicy flavors directly into the baking pan along with boneless chicken thighs. The red curry paste and chile pepper not only add potent taste to this dish, but they also increase metabolism, thin the blood, and contain heart-healthy antioxidants.

DAIRY-FREE, GRAIN-FREE

SERVES 4 | PREP TIME: 15 MINUTES, PLUS 1 HOUR TO MARINATE | COOK TIME: 1 HOUR

1 bunch fresh cilantro, washed, stems separated and leaves chopped

3 tablespoons crunchy peanut butter

1½ tablespoons Thai red curry paste

¼ cup lime juice

¼ cup soy sauce or tamari (or gluten-free substitute)

1 tablespoon brown sugar

1 tablespoon grated fresh ginger

1 (13-ounce) can full-fat coconut milk

8 boneless chicken thighs

½ cup roasted peanuts, chopped

1 red chile pepper, deseeded and finely sliced

1. To make the marinade, put the cilantro stems, peanut butter, red curry paste, lime juice, soy sauce, sugar, ginger, and coconut milk in a blender or food processor, and process until smooth.
2. Put the chicken in a glass bowl, coat with the marinade, and cover. Let marinate in the refrigerator at least 1 hour.
3. Preheat the oven to 350°F.
4. Place the chicken and marinade in a roasting pan.
5. Roast the chicken for 50 to 60 minutes, until it is golden and tender.
6. Before serving, garnish with the peanuts, chile pepper, and cilantro leaves. Serve extra sauce on the side, if desired.

SERVING TIP: Serve alongside steamed rice and Ginger-Spiked Baby Bok Choy (page 125).

HERB PROFILE: See Cayenne Pepper (page 31), Cilantro (page 54), and Ginger (page 49).

Nonna's Italian Meatballs

Everyone needs a tried-and-true comfort food recipe in their repertoire to pull out from time to time; these spicy herb- and garlic-laden meatballs are definitely one of mine. Garlic, oregano, and cayenne, all pungent herbs, make wonderful additions to cold-weather meals because they stimulate circulation, warm us up from the inside, enhance digestion of meats, and improve our resistance to infections.

NUT-FREE

MAKES 12 TO 16 MEATBALLS | PREP TIME: 20 MINUTES | COOK TIME: 1 HOUR 30 MINUTES

6 slices Italian bread, crusts removed and cubed

1 cup milk

1½ pounds ground beef or turkey

3 eggs, beaten

1 teaspoon salt

1 teaspoon freshly ground black pepper

½ cup chopped fresh parsley

1 to 2 tablespoons minced garlic

1 teaspoon dried oregano

½ teaspoon red pepper flakes

⅓ cup grated Pecorino Romano cheese

¼ cup plain dried bread crumbs

12 cups homemade or jarred marinara sauce

1. Preheat the oven to 400°F. Line a baking sheet with parchment paper.
2. Put the bread cubes into a small bowl and cover with the milk. Press the cubes down into the milk with the back of a spoon.
3. Put the meat in a large bowl and add the eggs, salt, pepper, parsley, garlic, oregano, pepper flakes, and cheese; mix gently to combine.
4. Using your hands, squeeze the milk out of the bread. Mix the soaked bread into the meat mixture. Discard the milk.
5. Add the bread crumbs to the meat mixture to absorb any excess moisture. Combine all of the ingredients well without overworking.

6. Divide the meat mixture in half. Each half should make 6 good-size meatballs or 8 smaller ones.
7. Scoop portions of the meat mixture out with a spoon and roll each meatball by hand.
8. Evenly space the meatballs on the prepared baking sheet.
9. Bake for 30 minutes, or until the meatballs have begun to brown.
10. Pour the marinara sauce into a large saucepan. Add the meatballs and simmer on medium-low for 1 hour or more.
11. Serve the meatballs and sauce over pasta or polenta.

COOKING TIP: These meatballs also hold up well in the slow cooker for a potluck crowd. Make them slightly smaller if you want to serve them with toothpicks or use in sandwich rolls.

MAKE-AHEAD TIP: I love to make a double batch and freeze them in quart-size containers for a quick meal on a busy day.

HERB PROFILE: See Garlic (page 59) and Oregano (page 65).

Summer Ratatouille with Chickpeas

This classic French summer stew is a great way to use garden overflow or seasonal vegetables from the market. Ratatouille was one of the first delightfully herb-infused meals I ever tasted at my friend Peggy's home nearly 40 years ago, and I've continued to enjoy this summer staple ever since. This slow cooker version is more convenient than cooking on the stove top. But if time allows, I do encourage you to make ratatouille on occasion doing just that. Add one ingredient at a time, slowly stirring, until the entire house is fragrant with antioxidant-rich basil, rosemary, and thyme.

DAIRY-FREE, GLUTEN-FREE, GRAIN-FREE, NUT-FREE, VEGAN

SERVES 4 TO 6 | PREP TIME: 20 MINUTES | COOK TIME: 4 TO 6 HOURS

6 tablespoons olive oil, divided

1 large onion, cut into 8 wedges

2 medium zucchini and/or yellow summer squash

1 medium eggplant

2 large sweet bell peppers, mixed colors

1 pound large flavorful tomatoes or 1 (28-ounce) can whole peeled tomatoes (I recommend San Marzano)

4 garlic cloves, coarsely chopped

1 (15-ounce) can chickpeas, drained

2 tablespoons tomato paste

1 teaspoon salt

1 teaspoon freshly ground black pepper

3 rosemary sprigs

6 thyme sprigs

¼ cup fresh basil leaves, torn

1. Heat 2 tablespoons of olive oil in a large skillet over medium-low heat. Add the onion wedges and cook until soft and light golden-brown, about 5 minutes. While the onions are sautéing, chop the rest of the vegetables.
2. Trim the ends off the zucchini and eggplant, cut into 1-inch cubes, and place in the slow cooker.
3. Trim and core the bell peppers, cut into 1-inch pieces, and add to the slow cooker.
4. Core the tomatoes, cut into 1½-inch pieces, and add to the slow cooker.
5. Add the garlic and chickpeas to the slow cooker.

6. When the onions are light golden brown, add the tomato paste to the pan, and stir to coat the onions. Transfer the onion mixture to the slow cooker. Add 2 tablespoons of olive oil, salt, and pepper and stir to coat all of the vegetables.
7. Strip the leaves from the stems of rosemary and thyme, and sink the herbs into the vegetables. Discard the stems.
8. Cover the slow cooker and cook until the vegetables are tender, about 4 hours on high or 6 hours on low.
9. When ready to serve, ladle the ratatouille into individual bowls, stir in the basil, and drizzle with more olive oil.

SERVING TIP: Serve with crusty bread or over rice or polenta. Any leftovers can be eaten cold with a drizzle of balsamic vinegar or used as a pizza topping. It always tastes better when the flavors have had ample time to mingle.

ROSEMARY

Fresh or dried leaf

SAFETY CONSIDERATIONS: Avoid during pregnancy in more than culinary amounts

TASTE/ACTIVITY: SPICY/WARM/DRY

PROPERTIES: Antidepressant, antioxidant, carminative, cerebral tonic, cholagogue, expectorant

USES: Relieves gas, bloating, and nausea; prevents oxidative damage; promotes circulation to the brain; allieviates mental fog and depression

SUGGESTED PREPARATIONS: Compound butter, culinary spice, infused oxymel, infused vinegar, tea

ESPECIALLY GOOD FOR: BRAIN HEALTH

There is a romantic adage that says, "Rosemary is for remembrance." In fact, this herb has been studied extensively in Europe in relation to its impressive antioxidative qualities and their impact on the brain. It is a cerebral tonic, improving circulation to the brain. It also improves memory, concentration, and cognitive function; and it can ease depression in the elderly. The superior antioxidants in rosemary protect the brain and blood vessels.

Classic Beef Stew

This slow-cook recipe is absolutely foolproof for creating great-tasting comfort food every single time. Achieving tender cubes of beef and pan-seared gravy does take some time, but it's well worth the effort. This classic beef stew uses red wine as well as fresh thyme, which provides one of the highest antioxidant concentrations of any herb and helps lower oxidative stress load in the body.

DAIRY-FREE, NUT-FREE

SERVES 4 | PREP TIME: 30 MINUTES | COOK TIME: 1 HOUR 30 MINUTES

1½ pounds boneless beef chuck, cubed

1 teaspoon salt

1 teaspoon freshly ground black pepper

2 tablespoons olive oil, plus more if needed

1½ cups diced yellow onion

3 tablespoons flour

1 cup red wine

2 cups water

3 garlic cloves, minced

3 bay leaves

6 thyme sprigs, stems removed (or 1 teaspoon dried)

2 cups new potatoes

4 or 5 carrots, cut at an angle into 1-inch-thick pieces

1. Preheat the oven to 450°F.
2. Pat the beef cubes dry with paper towels and season well with the salt and pepper.
3. In a heavy-bottomed, ovenproof pot with a tight-fitting lid, heat the olive oil over medium-high heat.
4. When the oil is very hot, carefully add half of the beef cubes, being careful not to crowd the pan.
5. Allow the beef to form a dark brown crust before turning, about 5 minutes. This crust will give deep flavor to the stew.
6. When the cubes are nicely browned on all sides, transfer to rest in a bowl.
7. Repeat the browning process with the other half of the beef, adding more oil to the pot if needed.
8. Set all of the browned meat aside in the bowl.
9. If the pan looks dry, add a little more oil and add the onion. Cook, stirring often, for 5 minutes.

〉〉〉〉〉〉

10. Add the flour to the cooked onions and stir to coat completely.
11. Add the red wine and water to the pot. Scrape up any browned bits on the bottom with a spatula.
12. Whisk continuously over medium heat until the liquid is thick and bubbling, about 5 minutes.
13. Add the beef cubes and juices from the bowl. Add the garlic, bay leaves, and thyme into the pot, and stir until thick and bubbly.
14. Immediately cover with a large piece of heavy-duty aluminum foil, carefully pressing the foil down onto the top of the stew and against the inside of the pot, sealing it tightly around the rim. This keeps the steam inside the stew and tenderizes the beef.
15. Cover the pot with the lid and slide it into the hot oven. Allow to braise for 1 hour and 30 minutes.
16. Meanwhile, in a large saucepan filled with water, and boil the potatoes and carrots until just tender, about 20 minutes.
17. Remove from heat, drain the water and keep the vegetables in the hot pan until the beef is finished.
18. Remove the pot from the oven after 1 hour and 30 minutes. Carefully remove the lid and foil, and stir in the vegetables. Discard the bay leaves. Serve hot.

SERVING TIP: This hearty meal needs little in the way of sides, but my choice would be to add a bitter leafy green vegetable, such as kale or collards, and some warm crusty bread.

SUBSTITUTION TIP: If you'd like to change up the taste of this stew, swap out the thyme and bay leaves in favor of a few tablespoons of spicy curry powder (containing turmeric) while sautéing the onions.

HERB PROFILE: See Thyme (page 97) and Turmeric (page 147).

THYME

Fresh or dried leaf

SAFETY CONSIDERATIONS: Avoid during pregnancy in more than culinary amounts

TASTE/ACTIVITY: SPICY/WARM/DRY

PROPERTIES: Antibacterial, antifungal, antioxidant, antiseptic, antispasmodic, antitussive, antiviral, aromatic carminative, bronchodilator, circulatory stimulant, decongestant, diaphoretic, expectorant, emmenagogue

USES: Aids digestion; treats congestion and wet coughs; stimulates circulation

SUGGESTED PREPARATIONS: Compound butter, culinary herb, infused honey, infused oxymel, infused syrup, infused tea, infused vinegar, inhalation steam

ESPECIALLY GOOD FOR: COUGHS, COLDS AND FLU

Thyme acts as an expectorant to help break down and expel mucus in the lungs due to bronchitis. It also acts as an antispasmodic in the case of an irritable tickle or asthmatic cough; helpful for sinusitis, tonsillitis, and pneumonia.

Stir-Fry with Chicken and 3 Cabbages

This quick stir-fry uses three beneficial *Brassica* genus members. The cabbage family pro-vides anti-inflammatory, detoxification, and anticancer benefits, as well as lots of vitamin C. Cruciferous vegetables naturally pair well with the pungent taste of ginger, garlic, and onions, and as a bonus, ginger increases and aids digestion. To make this entrée vegetarian, simply swap out the chicken for a 12-ounce block of tofu and omit the fish sauce.

DAIRY-FREE, GLUTEN-FREE, NUT-FREE

SERVES 4 | PREP TIME: 10 MINUTES | COOK TIME: 30 MINUTES

1 tablespoon coconut oil, plus 1 teaspoon

1 pound chicken breast, cut into bite-size pieces

½ teaspoon salt

½ teaspoon freshly ground black pepper

1 teaspoon grated fresh ginger

2 cups sliced Napa cabbage

1 cup sliced purple cabbage

2 cups baby kale

1 large carrot, peeled and cut at an angle into ¼-inch-thick slices

2 tablespoons water

2 garlic cloves, minced

1 teaspoon fish sauce

3 tablespoons tamari

1 teaspoon sesame oil

Juice of ½ lime

1 teaspoon sesame seeds

1. In a large skillet or wok, heat 1 tablespoon of coconut oil over high heat.
2. Add the chicken and sprinkle with the salt and pepper.
3. Cook for 3 minutes on each side, then transfer the chicken and its juices to a bowl.
4. Place the pan back over high heat and add the remaining 1 teaspoon of coconut oil.
5. Add the ginger, Napa cabbage, purple cabbage, baby kale, and carrot and cook for 2 minutes, stirring frequently.
6. Add the water, garlic, fish sauce, tamari, sesame oil, and lime juice, then return the chicken to the pan.
7. Stir to combine. Cook for 2 more minutes, stirring frequently.
8. Sprinkle with the sesame seeds and serve over steamed rice.

SUBSTITUTION TIP: Feel free to substitute any of your favorite cruciferous vegetables. Shredded Brussels sprouts, broccoli, and collard greens all work well in this recipe.

HERB PROFILE: See Ginger (page 49).

Pasta with Prosciutto and Peas

A handful of fresh mint and lemon zest brighten up this classic pasta pairing of ham and peas in cream sauce. We don't indulge in this kind of comfort food every day, but if there happens to be any smoky bits of leftover ham in the refrigerator, this dish is the first thing that comes to mind. Don't skimp on the hefty measures of black pepper, lemon, and mint; they all help activate the digestive process.

NUT-FREE, QUICK

SERVES 4 | PREP TIME: 10 MINUTES | COOK TIME: 15 MINUTES

1 pound fettuccine

2 tablespoons extra-virgin olive oil

½ onion, thinly sliced

4 ounces prosciutto, cut into thin ribbons

1 cup heavy cream

1 teaspoon freshly ground black pepper

⅛ teaspoon freshly grated nutmeg

1½ cups peas, fresh or frozen

½ cup grated Parmesan cheese, divided

½ cup chopped fresh mint, divided

1 teaspoon grated lemon zest

1 teaspoon freshly squeezed lemon juice

1. Bring a large pot of well-salted water to a boil and cook the fettuccine according to package directions until al dente. Drain, reserving ½ cup of the pasta cooking water.

2. While the pasta is cooking, heat the oil in a 12-inch skillet over medium-high heat. Add the onion to the skillet and cook, stirring, until translucent, about 3 minutes. Add the prosciutto ribbons and cook, stirring, until heated through and showing some brown bits, about 1 minute.

3. Add the heavy cream, black pepper, and nutmeg and bring to a simmer. Add the peas and reduce the heat to medium-low. Simmer, stirring often, until the peas are cooked through, about 5 minutes. Remove the skillet from the heat.

4. Add the cooked pasta to the sauce, along with half of the cheese and half of the mint. Add the lemon zest and juice.

5. Add some of the reserved pasta water, if needed, to thin the sauce.

6. Divide among 4 plates and top with the remaining cheese and mint.

SUBSTITUTION TIP: Feel free to swap pancetta, bacon, or ham for the prosciutto, and swap out the peas for asparagus if it is in season.

HERB PROFILE: See Mint (page 73).

Chili Cod Tacos with Lime Crema

Warm, soft corn tortillas are the perfect pocket for almost any quick meal at our house. This cod is seasoned with a blend of pungent spices that stimulate circulation and enhance digestion. Add in some crunchy raw vegetables, balance the heat with a cooling lime crema, and you have a very satisfying meal worthy of guests. For a vegetarian option, these same pungent spices can be added to black beans, warmed on the stove top, and served family style along with the rest of your taco sides.

GLUTEN-FREE, NUT-FREE, QUICK

SERVES 4 | PREP TIME: 15 MINUTES | COOK TIME: 15 MINUTES

½ cup sour cream

Zest of ½ lime

Juice of 1½ limes, divided

Dash cumin, plus ½ teaspoon

Dash garlic powder

2 tablespoons olive oil

2 pounds fresh cod fillets, preferably wild-caught

2 tablespoons unsalted butter

1 teaspoon chili powder

½ teaspoon dried oregano

½ teaspoon salt

16 (5-inch) soft corn tortillas

¼ head purple cabbage, thinly sliced

2 tomatoes, diced

2 avocados, pitted, peeled, and diced

1. Preheat the oven to 450°F.
2. Make the lime crema. In a small bowl, combine the sour cream, lime zest, juice of ½ lime, dash of cumin, and garlic powder. Cover and refrigerate until serving time.
3. Coat the bottom of a roasting pan with the olive oil and place the fish fillets in the pan.
4. Melt the butter in small saucepan and add the chili powder, oregano, ½ teaspoon cumin, salt, and the remaining juice of 1 lime. Stir to combine.
5. Brush the butter mixture over the cod and bake for 12 to 15 minutes, depending on the thickness of the fish, until it is opaque and flakes easily.
6. Wrap the stack of corn tortillas in two dampened paper towels, and then in aluminum foil.
7. During the last 5 minutes of cooking, place the wrapped tortillas in the oven to warm.
8. Arrange the cabbage, tomatoes, and avocados on a serving plate.
9. Remove the tortillas from the oven and transfer to a serving plate. Keep warm.

〉〉〉〉〉〉

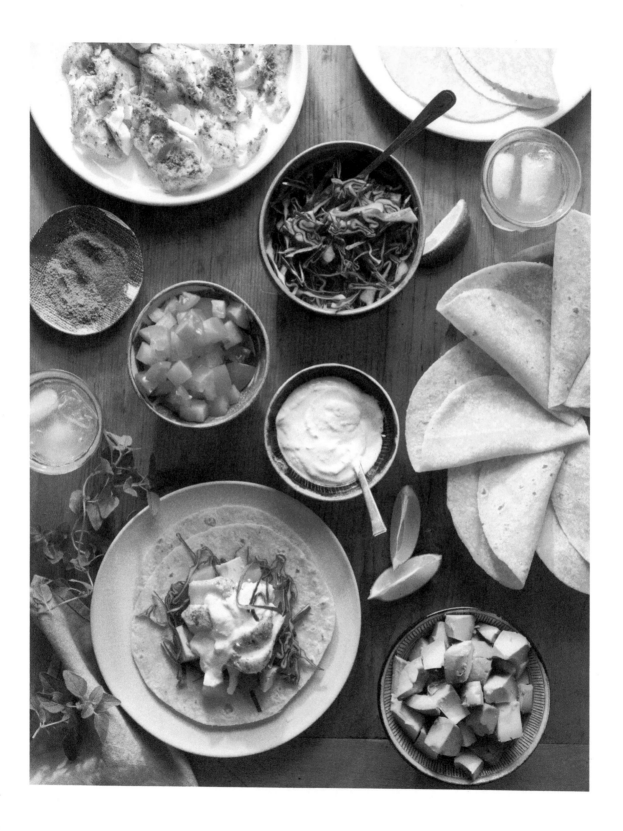

10. Remove the fish from the oven and break into 8 portions using the edge of a spatula, and transfer to a serving plate.
11. Serve the taco components family style, so that guests can fill their own warm tortillas with the fish and vegetables, and top with lime crema.
12. This recipe will make 8 tacos using 2 corn tortillas each.

SUBSTITUTION TIP: Cod and avocado provide some beneficial omega-3 fatty acids, but substituting salmon would boost it threefold!

HERB PROFILE: See Cayenne Pepper (page 31), Cumin (page 45), and Oregano (page 65).

Spanish Rice Zucchini Boats

Even if you don't have zucchini on hand, the Spanish rice tastes delicious enough to eat on its own. The cumin and oregano give this dish a bit of warming spice that aids in digestion. Feel free to add pungent Sriracha or cayenne pepper if you like it with an extra kick.

DAIRY-FREE, GLUTEN-FREE, NUT-FREE, VEGAN

SERVES 4 | PREP TIME: 10 MINUTES | COOK TIME: 30 MINUTES

Olive oil, for greasing, plus 1 tablespoon

2 medium zucchini, halved lengthwise

½ onion, chopped

½ red bell pepper, seeded and chopped

3 garlic cloves, minced

½ teaspoon cumin

½ teaspoon dried oregano

½ teaspoon paprika

½ teaspoon salt

½ teaspoon freshly ground black pepper

½ cup cooked rice

1 (15-ounce) can black beans, drained and rinsed

1½ cups prepared enchilada sauce

1 cup shredded vegan cheese (optional)

1. Preheat the oven to 400°F.
2. Lightly oil a 9-by-13-inch baking dish.
3. Using a teaspoon, scoop out the zucchini seeds and surrounding flesh so that a ¼-inch-thick shell remains.
4. In a skillet over medium heat, add 1 tablespoon of olive oil, the onion and pepper, and sauté for 5 minutes. Add the garlic, cumin, oregano, paprika, salt, and pepper, and cook for another minute.
5. Add the rice and black beans, and cook for an additional 3 minutes, until heated through. Remove from the heat.
6. Divide the rice mixture evenly between the zucchini halves and place them in the greased baking dish.
7. Top the zucchini evenly with the enchilada sauce.
8. Top with the shredded cheese, if using, and bake for 30 minutes.
9. Remove from the oven and let rest 5 minutes before serving.

SERVING TIP: This recipe can easily stand alone as a complete main dish without the zucchini. Or serve it with a side salad or steamed vegetable of your choosing.

HERB PROFILE: See Cumin (page 45), Garlic (page 59), and Oregano (page 65).

Quick Pad Thai

Making pad Thai simply requires a bit of chopping while the rice noodles soak and the shrimp sear. The cook time is only 15 minutes. While this recipe calls for shrimp, you can substitute tofu or chicken if you like. With any of the proteins you choose, the accompanying onion, garlic, ginger, and red pepper flakes provide a pungent taste that increases circulation, as well as warming, drying activity in the case of sinus or lung congestion.

DAIRY-FREE, QUICK

SERVES 4 | PREP TIME: 15 MINUTES | COOK TIME: 15 MINUTES

8 ounces pad Thai noodles
(wide rice noodles)

3 eggs

Salt

5 tablespoons fish sauce

5 tablespoons sugar (preferably coconut
sugar or brown sugar)

5 tablespoons rice wine vinegar

1 tablespoon soy sauce or tamari

2 tablespoons coconut oil, divided

8 ounces large shrimp, cleaned

1 small onion, minced

4 scallions, thinly sliced on the diagonal

3 or 4 garlic cloves, chopped

2 teaspoons chopped fresh ginger

1 (4-ounce) package fresh mung
bean sprouts

½ teaspoon red pepper flakes

½ cup peanuts, chopped, plus more
for garnish

1 lime, quartered

1. Place the rice noodles in a shallow baking dish and cover them with boiling water for 5 to 7 minutes. Drain and set aside.
2. In a small bowl, whisk the eggs with a fork and season with salt. Set aside.
3. In another small bowl, mix the fish sauce, sugar, rice vinegar, and soy sauce. Set aside.
4. Heat 1 tablespoon of coconut oil in a deep skillet or wok over medium-high heat. Sear the shrimp on both sides, 1 to 2 minutes. Set aside in a bowl.
5. Gather your bowls around the stove. In the same skillet or wok, heat the remaining 1 tablespoon of the coconut oil over medium heat. Add the onion, scallions, garlic, and ginger. Cook a few minutes, stirring, until golden and fragrant.

6. Make a well in the center of the pan and add the whisked eggs. With a spatula, scramble the eggs quickly, breaking them apart into little bits as you incorporate the onion, scallions, garlic, and ginger.
7. Immediately add the drained noodles and toss with the egg mixture, stirring and flipping constantly for a few minutes, until the noodles become soft and pliable.
8. Add the fish sauce mixture and the shrimp. Turn and toss the noodles for a few more minutes. (The fish smell will dissipate.)
9. Add the mung bean sprouts, red pepper flakes, and peanuts.
10. Divide among 4 plates.
11. Garnish with additional chopped peanuts and lime wedges.

INGREDIENT TIP: Pad Thai rice noodles are sold in the ethnic or Asian section of the grocery store, but if you can't find them, regular fettuccine noodles are a good substitute.

HERB PROFILE: See Cayenne Pepper (page 31), Garlic (page 59), and Ginger (page 49).

"The Greek" Lamb Burger with Feta Cheese and Tzatziki

Our family so enjoys the pungent flavors of the Greek Isles: lemon, garlic, rosemary, dill, and mint. These tastes are all showcased here in our favorite lamb burger recipe featuring carminative herbs known to aid digestion. Allowing the patties to rest in the fridge before cooking lets the flavors permeate.

NUT-FREE

SERVES 4 | PREP TIME: 20 MINUTES, PLUS 15 MINUTES TO CHILL AND REST THE BURGERS
COOK TIME: 10 MINUTES

1 pound ground lamb

2 tablespoons crushed dried mint

2 tablespoons minced fresh rosemary

2 garlic cloves, minced

½ teaspoon salt

½ teaspoon freshly ground black pepper

1 tablespoon olive oil

4 soft hamburger buns

4 romaine lettuce leaves

4 slices tomato

4 tablespoons crumbled feta cheese

½ cup tzatziki sauce, prepared or homemade (see page 74 for recipe)

1. In a large bowl, combine the lamb, dried mint, fresh rosemary, garlic, salt, and pepper.
2. Using your hands, gently mix the ingredients together; do not overmix.
3. Form the mixture into four patties. Place on a plate and cover with plastic wrap.
4. Refrigerate for 15 minutes while making the tzatziki sauce, if not using prepared.
5. Bring the burgers to room temperature. Heat a skillet over medium-high heat.
6. Add the olive oil to the hot pan, place the burgers in the pan, and cook for 4 minutes per side for medium-rare.
7. While the burgers are cooking, toast the buns cut-side down on a large griddle or skillet until lightly browned, about 3 minutes.

8. Remove the buns from the heat and place 1 lettuce leaf, 1 tomato slice, and 1 tablespoon of feta onto each bun bottom.

9. Top the bottom half of the buns with a lamb burger and 2 tablespoons of tzatziki. Cover with the top half of the bun and serve warm.

INGREDIENT TIP: You can find grass-fed ground lamb in the meat section of most grocery stores. All grass-fed meats and dairy products contain very high levels of CLA (conjugated linolenic acid), which is shown to reduce the risk of heart disease and cancer.

HERB PROFILE: See Rosemary (page 94), Mint (page 73), and Garlic (page 59).

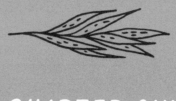

CHAPTER SIX

SNACKS AND SIDES

Some of these recipes reflect my early attempts to introduce medicinal herbs and spices into my young children's diets without raising too much suspicion on their part. When cold and flu season was bearing down, I made great bowls of garlicky hummus or pesto slathered on toast. As their tastes matured, I gave them lots of antiviral herbs chopped right into buttery mashed potatoes. I can happily report my kids have grown up into adults with great taste in food, in part thanks to these family-favorite dishes.

Sweet and Savory Nuts with Three Herbs

This potent trio of aromatic antioxidant and anti-inflammatory herbs packs a wallop in taste, protein, and medicinal value. Nuts are a great source of omega-3 fatty acids, but moderation is still key as they are an even bigger source of omega-6 fatty acids, which when consumed in large amounts can cause inflammation in the body.

GLUTEN-FREE, GRAIN-FREE, VEGETARIAN

SERVES 4 | PREP TIME: 10 MINUTES, PLUS 1 HOUR TO COOL | COOK TIME: 20 MINUTES

3 tablespoons unsalted butter

¼ cup maple syrup

Pinch ground cayenne pepper

2 cups mixed nuts (almonds, hazelnuts, walnuts, and pistachios)

½ teaspoon sea salt

1½ teaspoons freshly ground black pepper

1 teaspoon minced fresh sage

1 teaspoon minced fresh rosemary

1 teaspoon minced fresh thyme

1. Preheat the oven to 325°F.
2. In a small saucepan, heat the butter, maple syrup, and cayenne pepper over low heat until the butter is melted.
3. Add the mixed nuts and toss with a spoon until evenly coated.
4. Line a baking sheet with parchment paper; spread the nuts over it evenly.
5. Bake for 20 minutes or until most of the liquid has evaporated.
6. Remove from the oven, and immediately season with the salt, pepper, sage, rosemary, and thyme, stirring to coat the nuts.
7. Let the nuts cool for at least 1 hour before serving.

MAKE-AHEAD TIP: These are easy to make ahead when you have a few minutes to spare on the weekend. They'll make great snacks in lunches in the days ahead. Store in an airtight container in the refrigerator and consume within a week.

HERB PROFILE: See Thyme (page 97), Rosemary (page 94), Sage (page 111), and Cayenne Pepper (page 31).

SAGE

Fresh or dried leaf

SAFETY CONSIDERATIONS: Do not use during pregnancy or while breastfeeding (it will dry up and stop the flow of breast milk when used on a regular basis). Due to its drying activity, sage should not be used long-term by those who suffer from constipation, or dry cough, dry skin, hair, or eyes.

TASTE/ACTIVITY: SPICY/SLIGHTLY BITTER/WARM/DRY

PROPERTIES: AAntibacterial, anti-inflammatory, antioxidant, antiseptic, aromatic carminative, diaphoretic, expectorant

USES: Combats colds and flu, fever with chills, sore throat, hoarseness, sinus congestion, sinus infections, postnasal drip, and intestinal flu; as a tea/gargle treats mouth ulcers, gingivitis; soothes the mouth post dental surgery; relieves diarrhea, gas, and bloating

SUGGESTED PREPARATIONS: Compound butter, culinary herb, infused oxymel, infused syrup, infused vinegar, tea

ESPECIALLY GOOD FOR: COLD AND FLU RELIEF

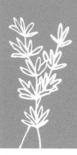

Sage is an herb most commonly used for cold and flu symptoms, particularly for red, painful sore throats; laryngitis, tonsillitis, and strep throat; drying up mucus in the sinuses and postnasal drip. Sage can also be used as an effective expectorant. As a diaphoretic, a cup of hot sage tea will bring on a good sweat, which is beneficial for detoxing.

Omega-3 Deep-Sea Pâté

Small, fatty, cold-water fish, such as sardines and mackerel, provide an abundance of beneficial omega-3 fatty acids, which may help lower blood pressure and triglycerides, and reduce the likelihood of heart attack and stroke. The American Heart Association recommends eating wild-caught fish two times per week, an easy goal when you have this recipe on hand.

GLUTEN-FREE, GRAIN-FREE, NUT-FREE

SERVES 4 | PREP TIME: 15 MINUTES, PLUS 2 HOURS TO CHILL

---

8 tablespoons (1 stick) unsalted butter, at room temperature and cut into large cubes

1 (4.4-ounce) can wild-caught, skinless, boneless sardines in olive oil, drained

1 (4.4-ounce) can wild-caught, skinless, boneless mackerel in olive oil, drained

3 tablespoons minced shallots (about 1 large shallot)

1 scallion, white and green parts, minced

3 tablespoons finely chopped parsley, plus more for garnish

3 to 4 teaspoons grated horseradish

1 tablespoon freshly squeezed lemon juice

½ teaspoon salt

½ teaspoon freshly ground black pepper

1. Combine the butter, sardines, mackerel, shallots, scallion, parsley, horseradish, lemon juice, salt, and pepper in a food processor and process until smooth and uniform in texture.
2. Transfer the pâté to serving dish. Cover and refrigerate for a minimum of 2 hours.
3. Garnish with additional parsley and serve.
4. Serve on crostini or toasted rye bread.

INGREDIENT TIP: You may use prepared horseradish normally found in jars in the perimeter of the fresh fish department or in the dairy aisle; however, it's easy to find horseradish root in the produce section if you'd like to grind your own.

HORSERADISH

Fresh root, prepared condiment, dried wasabi powder

SAFETY CONSIDERATIONS: Avoid during pregnancy in more than culinary amounts. Horseradish may irritate gastric mucosa.

TASTE/ACTIVITY: PUNGENT/HOT/DRY

PROPERTIES: Decongestant, expectorant, pungent carminative

USES: Stimulates digestion; helps metabolize fatty meats; relieves congestion in sinuses from allergies, sinus infection, hay fever, pneumonia, coughs, colds, and flu; supports lung health

SUGGESTED PREPARATIONS: Cocktail sauce, compound butter, condiment with meats, in tomato juice, infused vinegar, wasabi paste with sushi

ESPECIALLY GOOD FOR: COLD AND FLU RELIEF

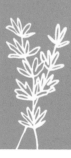

Horseradish helps thin and move out congestion in the sinuses and the lungs. It is strongly antibacterial in the case of sinus infections and cold, damp lung conditions, such as pneumonia, coughs, colds, and flu. For asthma, it can be used as a bronchodilator.

Spiced Pickled Red Beet Eggs

This recipe gives a sentimental nod to my native Pennsylvania German heritage. Red beet eggs are a traditional food served at many family gatherings. Vinegar and carminative spices are used to preserve and flavor the eggs, but the sour and spicy tastes are known to stimulate the appetite and help the body digest fats and heavy meats. You will need a quart-size wide-mouth jar for this recipe.

DAIRY-FREE, GLUTEN-FREE, GRAIN-FREE, NUT-FREE, VEGETARIAN

MAKES 6 EGGS | PREP TIME: 15 MINUTES, PLUS 36 HOURS TO PICKLE | COOK TIME: 45 MINUTES

FOR THE CARMINATIVE PICKLING SPICE BLEND

6 (3-inch) cinnamon sticks

6 tablespoons yellow mustard seeds

3 tablespoons whole allspice berries

2 tablespoons whole coriander seeds

2 teaspoons red pepper flakes (or less to taste)

3 bay leaves, crumbled

20 whole cloves

FOR THE RED BEET EGGS

1 large red beet, peeled, trimmed, and roughly chopped

2 cups water

6 hard-boiled eggs, peeled

2 tablespoons Carminative Pickling Spice Blend

1 cup apple cider vinegar

1 red onion, sliced

⅓ cup sugar

½ teaspoon salt

½ teaspoon freshly ground black pepper

TO MAKE THE CARMINATIVE PICKLING SPICE BLEND

1. Place the cinnamon sticks in a paper bag and crack them into smaller pieces with a rolling pin.
2. Mix the cinnamon, mustard seeds, allspice berries, coriander, red pepper flakes, bay leaves, and cloves together in a small bowl.

TO MAKE THE RED BEET EGGS

1. In a medium saucepan, simmer the chopped beet in the water, covered, until tender, about 35 minutes. Drain, reserving 1 cup of the cooking water.
2. Place the eggs in a quart-size wide-mouth jar.
3. Put 2 tablespoons of pickling spices and cooked beets in the jar on top of the eggs.

4. In the same saucepan, bring the reserved beet water, vinegar, onion, sugar, salt, and pepper to a simmer. Cook until the sugar has dissolved and the onion is softened and translucent, about 5 minutes.
5. Remove from the heat and allow to cool for 10 minutes.
6. Pour the warm vinegar-onion mixture over the eggs, beets, and pickling spices in the jar, covering the eggs completely. Cover with a plastic lid. (Vinegar can corrode the metal lid on mason jars.)
7. Refrigerate. The eggs will be ready to eat in a few days. Store the remaining carminative pickling spice blend in a jar with a lid.

PREPARATION TIP: For consistently perfect hard-boiled eggs, put 6 large eggs in a medium saucepan and cover with water. Bring the water to a hard boil, then turn off the heat and let the eggs rest in the water for 10 minutes. Drain the eggs and run cold water over them to stop the cooking.

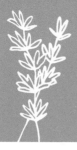

HERB PROFILE
CLOVES

Whole or ground dried unopened flower buds

SAFETY CONSIDERATIONS: Avoid during pregnancy in more than culinary amounts. Cloves can aggravate conditions of gastritis, ulcers, and irritable bowel syndrome.

TASTE/ACTIVITY: PUNGENT/HOT/DRY

PROPERTIES: Antibacterial, antiemetic, antioxidant, carminative, local anesthetic

USES: Stimulates digestion; relieves gas, nausea, intestinal bloating, cramping, and vomiting; treats bacterial diarrhea and food poisoning

SUGGESTED PREPARATIONS: Culinary spice, tea

ESPECIALLY GOOD FOR: DIGESTIVE RELIEF

Carminative herbs and spices help reduce the formation of gas bubbles created by gut bacteria in the digestive process. Carminatives also help eliminate intestinal spasms, burping, bloating, and flatulence.

Rosemary Feta Spread with Pita Points

This simple but sophisticated spread is piquant with sharp Mediterranean flavors. You can throw it together in moments if company comes, but if you can wait just a few hours for it to chill, the heady aromatic scent of rosemary permeates beautifully. Rosemary has one of the highest levels of antioxidants of any herb. Antioxidants help prevent the damage to cells caused by free radicals that contributes greatly to deteriorating illness and disease.

NUT-FREE, QUICK, VEGETARIAN

SERVES 4 | PREP TIME: 15 MINUTES

8 ounces feta cheese, crumbled

4 ounces cream cheese, softened

1 tablespoon grated lemon zest

1 tablespoon minced garlic

¼ cup minced fresh rosemary

½ teaspoon freshly ground black pepper

Olive oil, for garnish

Rosemary sprigs, for garnish

Pita bread, toasted and cut into triangles

1. Combine the feta, cream cheese, lemon zest, garlic, rosemary, and pepper in a medium bowl and blend well with a fork.
2. Transfer to a small serving bowl. Cover and refrigerate for a few hours, if you have time.
3. Drizzle with olive oil and garnish with rosemary sprigs. Serve with the pita points.

INGREDIENT TIP: It's best to use fresh rosemary in this dish, as the leaves are soft and very easy to chop. Dried rosemary can sometimes have an unpleasant mouthfeel because of its crunchy pine needle-like texture. Using it in soups and stews, where cooking will soften it, or grinding it into powder is a better use for the dried leaves.

HERB PROFILE: See Rosemary (page 94).

Hummus with Garlic

Hummus is a protein-packed bean dip that is the perfect vehicle for fresh, pungent garlic and was my original secret weapon against colds and flu when my children were small. Now this recipe is a family favorite just because it tastes so good. Use as much lemon juice as you like to make this dish bright with citrus taste and vitamin C.

DAIRY-FREE, GLUTEN-FREE, GRAIN-FREE, VEGAN

SERVES 4 | PREP TIME: 10 MINUTES, PLUS 3 HOURS TO CHILL

1 (15-ounce) can chickpeas, drained of most of the liquid (reserve 3 tablespoons for blending)

1 tablespoon tahini

Juice of 2 to 3 lemons

3 large garlic cloves

½ teaspoon salt

¼ to ⅓ cup olive oil

1. Put the chickpeas, reserved chickpea liquid, tahini, lemon juice, garlic, and salt in a food processor. Pulse to combine and make into a paste.
2. While the processor is running, slowly drizzle the olive oil through the top until the hummus reaches the texture you prefer.
3. Transfer to a bowl with a lid. Refrigerate for 3 hours to allow flavors to mingle.
4. Serve with fresh, crunchy crudités, like sliced carrots, celery, cucumbers, and peppers, or corn tortilla chips.

PREPARATION TIP: The food processor is the fastest, most convenient method to get a smooth-textured hummus, but remember, hummus has been made in the Middle East for centuries without modern appliances. Sometimes it's fun to mash everything up in a bowl using good old-fashioned elbow grease.

HERB PROFILE: See Garlic (page 59).

Golden Rice with Peas and Toasted Nuts

Why make plain rice when you can elevate your meal with golden rice? By adding the golden-hued Indian spice turmeric, you'll be imparting a pungent, earthy taste to your rice. You'll also step up your daily antioxidant intake, protect your liver, and lower overall systemic inflammation levels thanks to curcumin, turmeric's main chemical compound.

DAIRY-FREE, GLUTEN-FREE, VEGAN

SERVES 4 | PREP TIME: 15 MINUTES | COOK TIME: 30 MINUTES

2¼ cups water, divided

½ teaspoon salt, plus more for seasoning

1 cup basmati rice

3 tablespoons pine nuts or cashews (optional)

1 tablespoon coconut oil

¼ cup minced onions

¼ cup frozen peas

¼ teaspoon red pepper flakes

1 to 2 teaspoons Anti-Inflammatory Golden Paste (page 139)

Chopped fresh cilantro, for garnish

1. In a medium saucepan, bring 2 cups of water to boil and add the salt.
2. Add the rice and stir. Cover and reduce the heat. Simmer for 20 minutes or until the water is absorbed. Fluff and set aside.
3. Toast the nuts, if using, in a dry skillet for 3 to 5 minutes over medium heat until fragrant and golden. Set aside.
4. Heat the oil in the same skillet over medium heat. Add the onions, peas, and red pepper flakes. Cook for 5 minutes.
5. Reduce the heat to medium-low. Add the golden paste and the remaining ¼ cup of water to the skillet. Stir to blend.
6. Add the cooked rice and nuts to the skillet and stir until the rice is golden and the nuts and vegetables are evenly distributed. Season with salt to taste.
7. Heat through for 2 minutes.
8. Garnish with cilantro and serve immediately.

INGREDIENT TIP: Turmeric's vibrant yellow hue has been used to dye clothing for centuries. This means that turmeric can and will discolor every single thing it comes in contact with. Be sure to protect your countertop and clothing when cooking with turmeric.

HERB PROFILE: See Turmeric (page 147).

Barbecue Baby Lima Beans

The lowly lima bean boasts an enormous amount of fiber, which can lower blood sugar and cholesterol. Fiber combined with heart-protective cayenne and paprika make an awesome dietary combo that is perfect to take to the backyard barbecue. You can easily double this recipe for a crowd.

DAIRY-FREE, GLUTEN-FREE, VEGAN

SERVES 4 | PREP TIME: 10 MINUTES | COOK TIME: 25 MINUTES

2 tablespoons olive oil

1 cup chopped onion

2 garlic cloves, minced

8 ounces frozen baby lima beans

½ large green bell pepper, seeded and chopped

1 teaspoon smoked paprika

¼ teaspoon red pepper flakes

½ teaspoon dried oregano

1 cup crushed tomatoes

½ cup water

1 tablespoon freshly squeezed lime juice

¼ teaspoon salt

¼ teaspoon freshly ground black pepper

1. Heat a large skillet over medium-high heat.
2. Add the oil and onion; cook for 2 minutes, stirring frequently.
3. Add the garlic and continue cooking for another minute.
4. Add the lima beans, green pepper, paprika, and red pepper flakes, stirring constantly.
5. Once the spices have become aromatic, add the crushed tomatoes, water, and lime juice.
6. Bring to a low simmer, cover, and allow to steam for 10 minutes, stirring occasionally. Add the salt and pepper.
7. Remove the lid. Continue to simmer for 10 minutes longer, allowing some of the excess liquid to evaporate and the flavors to mingle before serving.

SERVING TIP: If you'd like to serve this dish to bacon-loving carnivores, you can stir in a few slices of cooked crumbled bacon during the last 10 minutes of cooking.

HERB PROFILE: See Cayenne Pepper (page 31).

Potato Gnocchi with Browned Sage Butter

Gnocchi is an Italian comfort food that I never made until about a year ago. I didn't realize what I was missing. The tiny potato-and-flour pasta pillows absorb whatever is captured in the little forked ridges. Here, gnocchi is a wonderful vehicle for the sage-infused sauce. Sage is a potent digestive carminative and antioxidant; crisping the herb in browned butter brings out its pungent aroma and taste.

QUICK, VEGETARIAN

SERVES 4 | PREP TIME: 5 MINUTES | COOK TIME: 20 MINUTES

3 cups cooked gnocchi (available in the frozen food aisle in 1-pound bags)

Olive oil

3 tablespoons butter

2 tablespoons finely slivered fresh sage

¼ cup pine nuts

3 garlic cloves, thinly sliced

Salt

Freshly ground black pepper

2 tablespoons finely chopped fresh parsley

1. Cook the gnocchi according to package directions. Drain, drizzle with a bit of olive oil, and keep warm.
2. Heat a large skillet over medium-low heat. Add the butter, allow to melt, and continue to heat slowly until you see some light brown solids forming in the pan, about 5 minutes. Add the sage and fry for about 1 minute, until it turns brown and crispy.
3. Reduce the heat to low; add the pine nuts and garlic. Stir constantly for an additional minute.
4. Remove the sage, pine nuts, and garlic from the pan with a slotted spoon and set aside.
5. Add the cooked gnocchi to the pan and cook for 5 to 7 minutes over medium heat, stirring occasionally, until brown and crispy. Season to taste with salt and pepper.

6. Turn off the heat. Add the sage, pine nuts, and garlic back into the pan, and stir to combine.

7. Sprinkle with fresh chopped parsley and serve.

SUBSTITUTION TIP: You can easily find fresh sage in the produce section of most grocery stores. The leaves are rather thick and leathery in texture, which lends itself well to the process of crisping in step 2. If you don't have access to the fresh leaves, you can substitute 1 teaspoon dried sage leaf, but reduce the time spent heating in brown butter to about 30 seconds.

HERB PROFILE: See Sage (page 111).

Roasted Winter Vegetables with Rosemary and Balsamic Glaze

A big tray of winter vegetables roasted with garlic and rosemary is a cold-weather comfort food beyond compare. Loaded with antiviral herbs, along with antioxidant-rich vegetables, this dish can help keep your immune system strong. Serve as a side to roast chicken or stir-fry into leftover golden rice and top with an egg for breakfast. This dish also makes a showstopping potluck offering with lots of fresh pine-scented rosemary sprigs added to the casserole.

DAIRY-FREE, GLUTEN-FREE, GRAIN-FREE, NUT-FREE, VEGAN

SERVES 4 | PREP TIME: 15 MINUTES | COOK TIME: 20 MINUTES

1 large sweet potato, washed (but not peeled) and cut into 8 chunks

1 red onion, peeled and cut into 8 wedges

2 beets, stem ends removed, washed (but not peeled) and quartered

2 cups Brussels sprouts, trimmed and halved

¼ cup chopped fresh rosemary

1 tablespoon olive oil

½ teaspoon salt

½ teaspoon freshly ground black pepper

1 large garlic bulb, excess paper covering removed, cut in half crosswise, and rubbed with olive oil on the cut ends

1 tablespoon balsamic glaze

1. Preheat the oven to 450°F. Line a baking sheet with parchment paper.
2. Place the sweet potato, onion, beets, and Brussels sprouts into a large bowl.
3. Add the rosemary, olive oil, salt, and pepper. Toss to coat all of the vegetables.
4. Arrange the vegetables on the prepared baking sheet.
5. Nestle the garlic bulb, cut-side up, among the chopped vegetables.
6. Bake for about 20 minutes or until fork-tender. Remove from the oven.

〉〉〉〉〉〉

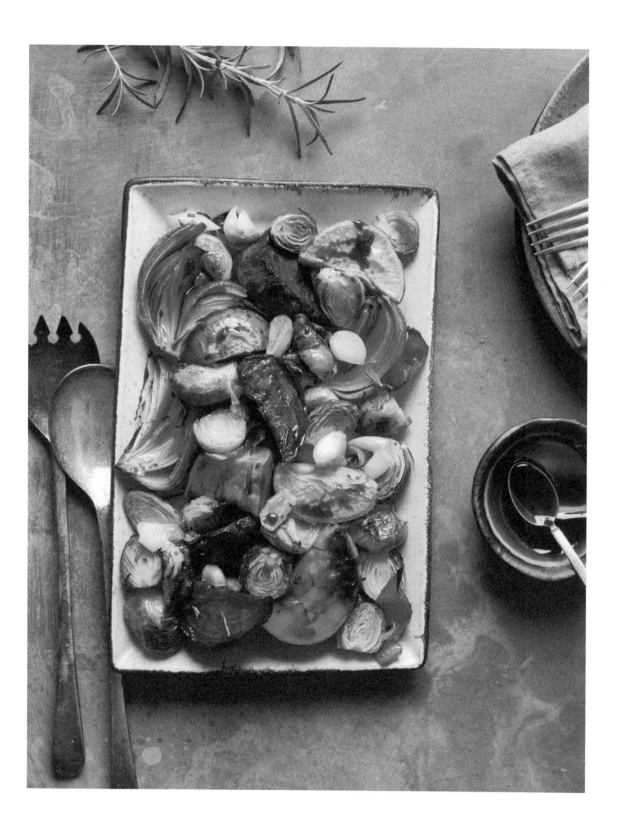

7. When cool enough to handle, remove the garlic and squeeze the roasted cloves out of the paper covering into the other vegetables. Stir to combine.
8. Drizzle with the balsamic glaze and serve immediately.

PREPARATION TIP: Balsamic glaze is a delicious sweet and sour condiment that you can find next to the vinegars in the grocery store. You can also make your own in a flash while the vegetables are roasting. Combine ½ cup balsamic vinegar and 3 tablespoons maple syrup, honey, or brown sugar in a saucepan over medium heat. When the mixture begins to bubble, reduce the heat to low and simmer until reduced by half, about 10 minutes. Remove from the heat. Will keep indefinitely in the refrigerator.

HERB PROFILE: See Rosemary (page 94).

Ginger-Spiked Baby Bok Choy

The pungent bite of ginger lends itself beautifully to the mild crunch of bok choy. This is a perfect accompaniment to roast pork, grilled fish, or tofu fried rice. Cruciferous vegetables, like bok choy, cabbage, broccoli, Brussels sprouts, cauliflower, collards, and arugula, are a medicinal food bomb. Multiple active compounds in these vegetables have been studied to show that they may not only prevent cancer but also protect against cell damage and inhibit tumor migration and tumor blood vessel formation.

DAIRY-FREE, GRAIN-FREE, NUT-FREE, QUICK, VEGAN

SERVES 4 | PREP TIME: 5 MINUTES | COOK TIME: 5 MINUTES

2 tablespoons olive oil

2 garlic cloves, minced

1 heaping teaspoon grated fresh ginger

2 pounds baby bok choy, washed and trimmed

1 tablespoon soy sauce

1 teaspoon toasted sesame oil

1 teaspoon sesame seeds

1. Heat the oil in a large sauté pan over medium heat. Add the garlic and ginger, and cook for 1 minute.
2. Cut the bok choy on an angle into 2-inch slices.
3. Add the bok choy, soy sauce, and sesame oil to the pan and cook, stirring constantly until the greens are wilted, the stalks are tender, and the condiments caramelize slightly, about 5 minutes.
4. Sprinkle the sesame seeds on top and serve immediately.

INGREDIENT TIP: Baby bok choy is sometimes available only seasonally in the produce section or at a farmers' market. These tiny cabbages are sweet, tender, and a joy to find. Full-size bok choy is readily available all year and may be substituted. It is equally delicious.

HERB PROFILE: See Ginger (page 49).

One-Pan Summer Squash Au Gratin with Thyme

A classic French au gratin dish combines potatoes with cream, cheeses, thyme, and bread crumbs: simple peasant food. Here, we substitute summer squash for potatoes, but the thyme leaves are really the star of the show. Thyme is an aromatic carminative herb that also has a potent amount of antiviral and antibacterial activity.

GLUTEN-FREE, GRAIN-FREE, NUT-FREE, VEGETARIAN

SERVES 4 | PREP TIME: 10 MINUTES | COOK TIME: 25 MINUTES

2 tablespoons butter

½ onion, very thinly sliced

2 large garlic cloves, minced

½ cup white wine, divided

½ cup heavy cream

½ teaspoon freshly ground black pepper

2 tablespoons fresh thyme
(or 1 tablespoon dried thyme)

¼ cup grated Parmesan cheese

1 zucchini, cut into ¼-inch-thick rounds

1 yellow squash, cut into ¼-inch-thick rounds

1 cup shredded Swiss cheese

½ cup gluten-free panko bread crumbs

1. Preheat the oven to 450°F.
2. Melt the butter in an ovenproof skillet over medium heat. Add the onion and cook until the edges start to brown, about 5 minutes.
3. Add the garlic and cook for 1 additional minute.
4. Add ¼ cup of white wine to deglaze the pan, scraping up any browned bits.
5. Add the cream, pepper, and thyme, and simmer until bubbly and starting to thicken. Slowly stir in the Parmesan cheese.
6. Add the zucchini and yellow squash, turning to coat all of the slices, and cook an additional 4 to 5 minutes.
7. Sprinkle with the Swiss cheese and bread crumbs, and bake for 10 to 15 minutes, until the cheese and bread crumbs are golden brown.

INGREDIENT TIP: Summer squash is an abundant, inexpensive choice at the height of the growing season. In fact, if you're a gardener, you're likely giving them away or looking for another way to serve them. The trick is to harvest or purchase squash that is young and tender. Older, larger squash can be tough and full of seeds. For a uniform look, choose zucchini and yellow summer squash that are the same size.

PREPARATION TIP: If you are using fresh thyme, you can easily strip the leaves from the stems by pulling them off in the direction of the woody end. It's so much quicker than chopping, and there's no need to chop the tiny leaves once you've stripped them from the stem; they are ready to use.

HERB PROFILE: See Thyme (page 97).

CHAPTER SEVEN

CONDIMENTS

This chapter features basic herbal preparations that you can make ahead and store in your pantry or refrigerator to use as needed. I'll describe how to infuse herbs into vinegars, syrups, and honeys to create delicious medicinal beverages, dressings, marinades, and sauces. I'll provide easy recipes for flavor-packed herb pestos and compound butters that can be immediately stirred into pastas, soups, and vegetables or conveniently frozen for later use. Make these recipes when the herbs are fresh and abundant, so you'll have a nicely stocked pantry to enhance your medicinal cooking all year round.

Basic Herb-Infused Vinegar

Herbal vinegars combine the nutritional properties of raw apple cider vinegar with the mineral and antioxidant-rich potential of herbs. These preparations not only provide delicious medicine; they are also the best medium (besides water) for extracting minerals from plants. Minerals are important for the health and proper functioning of bones, heart, blood vessels, nerves, brain, and immune system. I've included a few herbal vinegar variations to use in salad dressings and in marinades. For delicious drinking vinegars, see chapter 8 (page 141).

DAIRY-FREE, GLUTEN-FREE, GRAIN-FREE, NUT-FREE, VEGAN

MAKES 1 PINT | PREP TIME: 10 MINUTES, PLUS 3 TO 4 WEEKS TO INFUSE

1 cup chopped fresh herbs, or ⅓ cup dried herbs (see suggested herb combinations in tip)

2 cups raw apple cider vinegar

1. Fill a pint-size, wide-mouth mason jar with the fresh (or dried) aromatic herbs.
2. In a medium saucepan, warm the apple cider vinegar slightly over medium heat to the same temperature as just-right tea. Warming the vinegar (but not boiling it) will help jump-start the infusion process.
3. Pour the slightly warmed raw apple cider vinegar over the herbs and fill to within 1 inch of the top of the jar.
4. Cover the jar with a plastic screw-on lid or use several layers of plastic wrap (or wax paper) held in place with a rubber band. Vinegar will cause corrosion on a metal lid.
5. Label the jar with the name of the herb(s) and the date you made it. Mark your calendar 3 to 4 weeks ahead to remind yourself to strain the vinegar. Keep the jar out of direct sunlight. It is not necessary to refrigerate; on the counter is fine. Give it a good shake once or twice per week. You may notice that the vinegar changes color or takes on the aromatic quality of the herb. That's a good thing.
6. After 3 to 4 weeks, strain the vinegar into a clean jar and discard the herbs. Label and store in a kitchen cabinet.

INGREDIENT TIP: The preferred vinegar for culinary and medicinal herb infusions is organic raw apple cider vinegar. White distilled vinegar is made from grains and not the best for ingesting. However, it does make a wonderful inexpensive base for herb-infused cleaning vinegars. White vinegar also makes a great weed killer, if you happen to need one.

SUGGESTED HERBS (USE SINGLY OR IN COMBINATION):

» Oregano, basil, and chives
» Parsley, sage, rosemary, and thyme
» Chive blossoms, lavender flowers, and mint

TO USE: Make a very basic vinaigrette by combining ¼ cup herb-infused vinegar, ¾ cup olive oil, and salt and pepper to taste in a ½-pint mason jar. Cover and shake well. Store at room temperature. For more tang, add a tablespoon of prepared mustard and a pinch of sugar (or experiment with other seasonings).

HERB PROFILE: See Oregano (page 65), Basil (page 43), Mint (page 73), Parsley (page 82), Sage (page 111), Rosemary (page 94), Thyme (page 97), and Lavender (page 154).

Herbal Pantry Immune Vinegar

This pungent combination of herbs and other foods infused into vinegar is a traditional remedy for colds and flu. Make this in late summer to early fall so it's ready to use when you need it most. Simply add a tablespoon or two to a cup of hot water with honey to make an immune-stimulating tea at the first sign of a cold. Think of it as hot and spicy lemonade.

DAIRY-FREE, GLUTEN-FREE, GRAIN-FREE, NUT-FREE, VEGAN

MAKES 1 CUP | PREP TIME: 20 MINUTES, PLUS 3 TO 4 WEEKS TO INFUSE

1 tablespoon prepared horseradish

1 tablespoon chopped garlic

1 tablespoon chopped onion

1 tablespoon chopped fresh ginger

3 tablespoons dried elderberries

2 slices lemon and/or orange

½ teaspoon red pepper flakes

1 cup raw apple cider vinegar

1. Put the horseradish, garlic, onion, ginger, elderberries, lemon, and pepper flakes in a pint-size wide-mouth mason jar.
2. Add the vinegar.
3. Cover with a plastic lid or plastic wrap under a metal lid to avoid corrosion. Shake well.
4. Label the jar "Immune Vinegar" along with the date.
5. Let the immune vinegar infuse for 3 to 4 weeks, shaking the jar at least one time per week. Strain and decant the vinegar into a clean jar. Discard solids.

TO USE: Add 1 to 3 tablespoons of your finished immune vinegar to a cup of hot, steaming water. Adding a spoonful of honey to the hot water creates the perfect balance of heat and sweet. Sip hot at the first sign of a sniffle, chill, sore throat, or cough. Repeat as needed.

PREPARATION TIP: This recipe is eternally forgiving in its measurements. You can halve or double the ingredients as needed. Many people like to alter the recipe from one year to the next, adding more heat, garlic, or citrus. Some add a few tablespoons of honey right in. Make this immune tonic to your liking, and be sure to use it! It will warm you up, make you sweat, and may keep you healthy all winter long.

HERB PROFILE: See Horseradish (page 113), Garlic (page 59), Ginger (page 49), Elderberry (page 87), and Cayenne Pepper (page 31).

Basic Herb-Infused Syrup

Like Mary Poppins loves to tout: A spoonful of sugar helps the medicine go down! Herbal syrups can be used as a flavorful sweet addition to teas, sparkling water, fruit salad, and yes, even cocktails. They can also be used in a medicinal way, as in ginger syrup for nausea or antiviral elderberry syrup for fighting off a cold. See a few additional herbs suggested in the ingredients. See chapter 8 (page 141) for more recipes using herbal syrups.

DAIRY-FREE, GLUTEN-FREE, GRAIN-FREE, NUT-FREE

MAKES 2 CUPS | PREP TIME: 10 MINUTES | COOK TIME: 20 MINUTES, PLUS 1 HOUR TO STEEP

1 cup water

2 cups sugar

1 cup chopped fresh herbs, or ½ cup dried herbs (such as mint, ginger, lavender, rose petals, rose hips, elderberries)

1. Stir the water and sugar together in a small saucepan.
2. Turn the heat to medium-low and bring to a low simmer. Stir until the sugar has dissolved. Do not boil.
3. Add the herbs; cover and simmer on low for 20 minutes.
4. Turn off the heat. Cover and let steep at least 1 hour to overnight.
5. Strain the syrup into a clean jar; label and refrigerate. It should last a year in the refrigerator.
6. You may also seal it in a water bath canner if you want to store at room temperature.

TO USE: Add 1 to 2 teaspoons of your favorite herb-infused sweet syrup to flavor a mojito or plain sparkling water, or as a drizzle over fruit.

PREPARATION TIP: This recipe is based on the standard simple syrup preparation and contains quite a bit of sugar. In this case, sugar is used as a preservation method. Using the 2:1 sugar-to-water ratio will give your herbal syrup a longer shelf life in the refrigerator. Using a 1:1 sugar to water ratio will make it a little less sweet; however, the refrigerator shelf life may be substantially shorter.

HERB PROFILE: See Mint (page 73), Ginger (page 49), Elderberry (page 87), and Rose (page 159).

Basic Herb-Infused Honey

Infusing herbs into honey is another sweet way to enhance your medicinal cooking. Add to teas, fruit salads, marinades, desserts, and beverages. Be sure to support your local bee-keepers by purchasing their honey wherever possible. Some honeys available in large chain grocery stores are imported from China and of inferior quality.

DAIRY-FREE, GLUTEN-FREE, GRAIN-FREE, NUT-FREE, VEGETARIAN

MAKES 1 CUP | PREP TIME: 10 MINUTES | COOK TIME: 1 HOUR, PLUS 8 HOURS TO STEEP

1 cup local honey

½ cup chopped dried or wilted herbs, such as sage, rose petals, thyme, or lavender (see tip)

1. Gently heat the honey and herbs together in the top of a double boiler over medium-low heat. Cook for 1 hour, until the honey is runny and the herbs are fragrant. Do not boil.
2. Turn off the heat, cover, and allow to steep overnight.
3. The next morning, warm the honey just enough to facilitate straining.
4. When the honey is warm and runny, strain through a fine-mesh strainer held over a clean jar to capture the honey.
5. Wipe the jar, put on the lid, and label. Store at room temperature.

TO USE: You may use herb-infused honeys in the same way you would herbal syrups. However, because of its viscosity, honey is best incorporated into something warm, like hot tea, so that it dissolves. It will sink to the bottom of a cold drink.

INGREDIENT TIP: Using herbs with high moisture content may cause the honey to ferment or cause mold to form on exposed plant material. If you'd like to use fresh herbs, harvest them on a hot, dry day and allow the herbs to wilt for several hours on the countertop before chopping and mixing with honey. I have made herbal honeys successfully many times using fresh wilted rose petals, lavender buds, bee balm, sage leaf, anise hyssop, and even cayenne peppers.

HERB PROFILE: See Sage (page 111), Lavender (page 154), Rose (page 159), and Thyme (page 97).

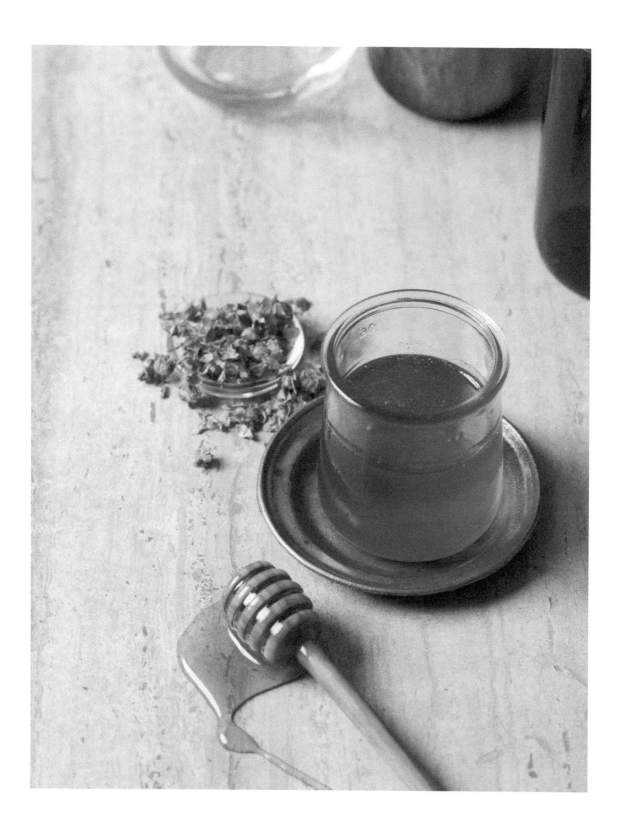

Basic Electuary

An electuary is an ancient method of combining honey and medicinal herbs to help mask the unpleasant taste of some herbs. Fortunately, in this recipe, we are blending only delicious, warming carminative spices. Carminatives aid digestion, stimulate circulation, and just happen to taste good doing it.

DAIRY-FREE, GLUTEN-FREE, GRAIN-FREE, NUT-FREE, VEGETARIAN

MAKES 2 CUPS | PREP TIME: 15 MINUTES | COOK TIME: 1 HOUR, PLUS 8 HOURS TO STEEP

1 teaspoon ground cloves

2 teaspoons ground coriander

2 teaspoons ground ginger

2 teaspoons freshly ground black pepper

2 teaspoons ground fennel

2 teaspoons ground nutmeg

1 tablespoon ground cardamom

1 tablespoon ground allspice

3 tablespoons ground cinnamon

¼ teaspoon ground cayenne

2 cups local honey

1. In a double boiler, stir the cloves, coriander, ginger, pepper, fennel, nutmeg, cardamom, allspice, cinnamon, and cayenne into the honey, and warm together over low heat for 1 hour, stirring often. Avoid heating the honey over 100°F, as this destroys its beneficial qualities. (Low and slow is the way to go!) Remove from the heat and allow to sit overnight.

2. The powdered spices will remain in the honey; they are not strained out. The finished electuary will be rich, dark, fragrant, and nearly paste-like in consistency.

3. Store in a clean, covered jar at room temperature. This is absolutely delicious stirred into a cup of black tea with cream for instant chai.

TO USE: You could eat this right off the spoon if so inclined! Adding a teaspoon or two stirred into tea or slathered on buttered toast is a fantastic way to use this medicinal food.

PREPARATION TIP: As a labor of cooking love, I enjoy using whole spices and powdering them myself in a coffee grinder, but you may use commercially prepared ground spices. If you do opt to grind them yourself, be very thorough; you want powder instead of crunchy little bits that might hurt your teeth.

HERB PROFILE: See Cloves (page 115), Ginger (page 49), Fennel (page 77), Cardamom (page 39), Cinnamon (page 35), and Cayenne Pepper (page 31).

Basic Compound Butter

A compound butter is a fancy name for softened butter into which chopped aromatic herbs have been incorporated. It's a perfect way to preserve the last bits of herbal greenery from the garden or the farmers' market at the end of the growing season. Herb-infused butters can be used on grilled meats, in rice, or on pastas. I love pulling herbal butters out of the freezer over the holidays. It's a satisfying way to impress your guests and introduce them to the flavorful benefits of herbs rich in antioxidants. This recipe is easily adapted to making larger batches and freezing.

GLUTEN-FREE, GRAIN-FREE, NUT-FREE, QUICK, VEGETARIAN

MAKES 8 TABLESPOONS | PREP TIME: 15 MINUTES

¼ cup finely minced aromatic and pungent herbs (such as thyme, garlic, rosemary, dill, chives or chive blossoms, parsley, or horseradish)

8 tablespoons (1 stick) butter, at room temperature

1. In a bowl, incorporate the herbs into the butter with a rubber spatula.
2. Scrape the finished compound butter onto a piece of parchment paper, wrap, and loosely roll into the shape of a log.
3. Twist the ends of the parchment to make a tight tube and refrigerate or put in a freezer bag and freeze until ready to use. Simply slice off coin-shaped pieces as needed.

TO USE: When you need to use it, pull the tube out of the freezer bag and thaw slightly. Using a sharp knife, cut off 1 tablespoon portions to serve with baked potatoes or winter squash, poached fish, grilled corn on the cob, or warm crusty bread.

SUBSTITUTION TIP: For a sweet-tasting compound butter, combine the butter with a few tablespoons of Dandelion Marmalade or the rose petal variation (page 46) or Basic Electuary (page 136).

HERB PROFILE: See Thyme (page 97), Garlic (page 59), Rosemary (page 94), Dill (page 75), Parsley (page 82), and Horseradish (page 113).

Basic Herbal Pesto with Basil

Made with fresh basil, pesto is a traditional herbal paste recipe from Genoa, Italy, that is stirred into warm pasta or rice. With a little imagination, we can substitute other aromatic, antioxidant-rich herbs to create a variety of flavor profiles for many dishes (see tip).

GLUTEN-FREE, GRAIN-FREE, QUICK, VEGETARIAN

MAKES 1 CUP | PREP TIME: 10 MINUTES

2 cups fresh basil leaves

2 or 3 large garlic cloves

½ cup grated Parmesan cheese

¼ cup pine nuts or walnuts

½ cup olive oil

1. Put the basil leaves, garlic, cheese, and nuts into the bowl of a food processor or blender.
2. Turn the processer on low. At the same time, drizzle the olive oil slowly into the opening at the top of the processor, until all of the ingredients are blended into a paste.
3. Store in a glass jar with a lid. To diminish the inevitable darkening of the pesto, drizzle a thin layer of olive oil over the top before storing in the refrigerator.

TO USE: Spoon a few tablespoons of this flavorful herb paste over hot pasta or rice and toss to distribute. Add a dollop of pesto to soups, stews, pizza, or fresh sliced tomatoes.

SUBSTITUTION TIP: For a vegan option, remove the cheese from the recipe or substitute vegan cheese. You may substitute any other culinary herb here for the basil. Rosemary pesto complements lamb or roasted potatoes; an oregano version is delicious on pizza.

FREEZING TIP: Herbal pesto freezes very well. I like to freeze individual portions in ice cube trays so I can take out whatever I need at a moment's notice.

HERB PROFILE: See Basil (page 43).

Anti-Inflammatory Golden Paste

Turmeric is a very popular anti-inflammatory herb that has been used for thousands of years in India and the Middle East. It was never taken as a supplement but always incorporated into daily cooking as a valuable healing spice. By using this golden paste, we can easily incorporate turmeric into our regular cooking rotation the way it is best absorbed in our bodies: with a healthy fat and black pepper.

DAIRY-FREE, GLUTEN-FREE, GRAIN-FREE, NUT-FREE, QUICK, VEGAN

MAKES ¾ CUP | PREP TIME: 5 MINUTES | COOK TIME: 10 MINUTES

½ cup organic ground turmeric

1 cup water

⅓ cup coconut oil

½ to 1 teaspoon freshly ground
    black pepper

1. Combine the turmeric and water in a small saucepan and stir constantly over low heat for 7 to 9 minutes. This will dissolve some of the grittiness of the powder.
2. Add the coconut oil and black pepper; stir until the oil has melted and is well integrated into the turmeric.
3. Store in a covered glass jar in the refrigerator for up to 4 weeks. Because coconut oil is liquid above 76°F, but solid when chilled, the golden paste will solidify in the refrigerator.

TO USE: Golden paste adds a warming and exotic flavor to vegetables, soups, egg and chicken dishes, creamy beverages, Classic Beef Stew (page 95), Golden Rice with Peas and Toasted Nuts (page 118).

INGREDIENT TIP: Turmeric is best absorbed and utilized in the body when ingested with a fat and accompanied by black pepper; golden paste combines all three ingredients.

HERB PROFILE: See Turmeric (page 147).

CHAPTER EIGHT

BEVERAGES

Beverages created with herbs are often a first introduction to medicinal cooking. They almost always taste and smell good, but that is just the beginning. Tea-making takes an act of slowing down, being present, choosing an herb, and waiting for water to boil. Once the steam-carrying volatile oils reaches your nose, the body and mind are close behind, anticipating and activating a healing response. Sipping aromatic beverages stirs a multitude of physiological responses, but the simple act of *creating it* is also nourishing to mind, body, and soul. Such is the magic of mindful medicinal cooking. There is so much here to delight your senses, from a soothing tisane to cooling iced teas, a pungent herbal cocktail, or a creamy rose lassi.

Tulsi Tisane

Tulsi is the Sanskrit name for the holy basil plant, which is native to India and has been a significant herb in Ayurvedic medicine for thousands of years. This herb is considered to uplift the spirit and chase away brain fog and muddled thinking caused by long-term stress, depression, menopause, and even brain injury. A tisane is simply an herbal tea (as opposed to a caffeinated black tea) that's as simple to make as pouring boiling water over dried herbs. If you find tulsi tea bags at the grocery store, it's surely worth experiencing. But if you have a place to plant your own, you will love its presence in your life, I guarantee it. Tulsi has earned its reputation as "liquid yoga" for a reason!

DAIRY-FREE, GLUTEN-FREE, GRAIN-FREE, NUT-FREE, QUICK, VEGAN

SERVES 1 | PREP TIME: 5 MINUTES, PLUS 15 MINUTES TO STEEP

1 cup boiling water

1 teaspoon dried holy basil/tulsi or
1 tablespoon chopped fresh

1. In a French press or mason jar, pour the boiling water over the herb.
2. Cover and steep for 15 minutes.
3. Strain the beverage. Inhale deeply; exhale deeply. Sip.

GROWING TIP: Like its culinary cousin, holy basil can grow wherever full sun and adequate water are provided. You may not find these plants readily available at your local garden center, but it is easy to start from seeds scattered on warm fertile soil. Check the Resources section (page 185) for recommended herbal seed and bulk herb suppliers.

HOLY BASIL

Fresh or dried leaf and flowers

SAFETY CONSIDERATIONS: Avoid during pregnancy and while breast-feeding in more than culinary amounts. Holy basil is generally considered safe but may potentiate anticoagulant and insulin medications.

TASTE/ACTIVITY: SPICY/SWEET/WARM/NEUTRAL

PROPERTIES: Adaptogen, antibacterial, antidepressant, antioxidant, antiviral, anxiolytic, carminative, galactagogue, immunomodulator, mild antispasmodic, neuroprotective, relaxing nervine

USES: Eases stress, mental fog, and mental exhaustion from chronic stress; supports homeostasis in the body

SUGGESTED PREPARATIONS: Infused tea, infused honey, infused syrup, infused vinegar, and infused oxymel

ESPECIALLY GOOD FOR: OVERALL WELL-BEING

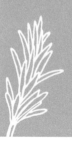

Adaptogens aren't used for treating a specific condition. Instead they support overall well-being by helping the body adapt to wide-ranging stressors, such as environmental and emotional stress, physical exhaustion, burning the candle at both ends, insomnia, or grief. Adaptogens work steadily but slowly over a long period of time to bring the mind and body back into balanced harmony. Holy basil is considered a sacred plant (also called tulsi) in India and is a wonderful adaptogen that's been used in Ayurvedic traditions for thousands of years.

HIBISCUS–LIME ICED TEA

Hibiscus flowers provide one of the most stunning shades of deep red in the entire food world, and this herb is a powerhouse of antioxidant-rich flavonoids and vitamin C. This also gives hibiscus its delicious tart taste. Paired with spearmint and lime, it makes a spectacular cooling iced tea for the summer months.

DAIRY-FREE, GLUTEN-FREE, GRAIN-FREE, NUT-FREE, VEGAN

SERVES 2 | PREP TIME: 5 MINUTES, PLUS 15 MINUTES TO STEEP AND 2 HOURS TO CHILL

3 cups water

2 tablespoons dried hibiscus flowers

1 tablespoons dried spearmint leaves

2 tablespoons sugar

2 tablespoons freshly squeezed lime juice

1. Bring the water to a boil in a medium saucepan.
2. Once boiling, add the dried hibiscus flowers and mint. Cover and remove from the heat.
3. Let the tea steep for 15 minutes.
4. Add the sugar and lime juice, and stir until the sugar is completely dissolved. Strain the herbs out of the tea.
5. Chill the tea in the refrigerator for at least 2 hours. Serve over ice with a slice of orange.

SOURCING TIP: Dried hibiscus flowers aren't generally available in regular grocery stores. Check the Resources section (page 185) for places to purchase these ruby-colored gems.

HIBISCUS

Dried calyces

SAFETY CONSIDERATIONS: Avoid in large quantities with prescription blood pressure medications

TASTE/ACTIVITY: SOUR/COOL/MOIST

PROPERTIES: Anti-inflammatory, antioxidant, demulcent, diuretic, anti-inflammatory

USES: Promotes heart health and lowers blood pressure

SUGGESTED PREPARATIONS: Infused syrups, infused vinegar, warm or iced tea

ESPECIALLY GOOD FOR: ANTIOXIDANTS

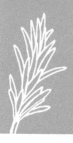

Hibiscus is loaded with vitamin C. Hibiscus flowers are a great source of antioxidants, which play a role in heart health and lowering blood pressure. It also has some diuretic qualities and is cooling and anti-inflammatory in nature.

Chai-Spiced Golden Milk

The main ingredient in this warming carminative recipe is turmeric. Turmeric contains curcumin, which is currently being studied for over 500 medicinal benefits. Curcumin must be combined with a full fat and black pepper to make it available to the cells in the body. This traditional Ayurvedic drink is not only a nutritional anti-inflammatory and anticancer powerhouse, it is remarkably delicious, as well. It is recommended that a mere ½ teaspoon of turmeric per day, prepared this way, is a substantial health boon. All of the ingredients can be adjusted for individual tastes and recipe doubled as desired.

GLUTEN-FREE, GRAIN-FREE, NUT-FREE, QUICK, VEGETARIAN

SERVES 1 | PREP TIME: 5 MINUTES | COOK TIME: 10 MINUTES

1 cup whole milk or unsweetened coconut, rice, or nut milk

1 generous teaspoon honey or maple syrup

1 teaspoon coconut oil

½ teaspoon organic ground turmeric

¼ teaspoon ground cardamom

Pinch ground ginger

Pinch ground cloves

Pinch ground allspice

Pinch freshly ground black pepper

½ teaspoon vanilla extract

1. Warm the milk, honey, and coconut oil in a small saucepan over low heat.
2. When the milk becomes warm, add the turmeric powder.
3. Whisk to dissolve any lumps. The milk will take on a rich, golden color.
4. Add the cardamom, ginger, cloves, allspice, pepper, and vanilla. Keep the pot on low heat for 3 additional minutes, until the spices are incorporated.
5. Pour into a mug and enjoy warm.

INGREDIENT TIP: See the recipe for Anti-Inflammatory Golden Paste (page 139) for more ways to use the super food, turmeric.

HERB PROFILE: See Turmeric (page 147), Cardamom (page 39), and Ginger (page 49).

TURMERIC

Fresh and ground dried rhizome; also known as curcumin in standardized supplement form (best to purchase certified organic)

SAFETY CONSIDERATIONS: Although turmeric is considered safe, some people may experience side effects, including nausea, diarrhea, or stomach upset. Due to its digestive stimulating activity, turmeric should be used cautiously with gastric reflux, stomach ulcers, hyperacidity, and pregnancy.

TASTE/ACTIVITY: SLIGHTLY PUNGENT/BITTER/WARM/DRY

PROPERTIES: Antibacterial, anti-inflammatory, antimutagenic, antioxidant, carminative, cholagogue, hepatoprotective, and tonic

USES: Relieves pain from arthritis, rheumatoid arthritis, and bursitis; treats inflamed bowel tissue, leaky gut, irritable bowel syndrome, Crohn's disease, colitis, diverticulitis, and liver disease; regenerates liver function; stimulates digestion and proper absorption of foods; kills *E. coli*, staph, and strep; lowers blood pressure, reduces LDL cholesterol levels, and reduces oxidative damage to blood vessels

SUGGESTED PREPARATIONS: The beneficial compounds in turmeric are not water soluble, so tea will have little to no activity. To obtain the best absorption of its active compound, curcumin, turmeric must be ingested with black pepper (which increases its absorption by 2,000 percent) and a fat, such as coconut oil, coconut milk, ghee, or avocado. Make into Anti-Inflammatory Golden Paste (page 139) and add to rice, eggs, soups, and curries. Note that turmeric is the main spice in curry powder so it may be used interchangeably in cooking.

ESPECIALLY GOOD FOR: REDUCING INFLAMMATION

Turmeric is a strong anti-inflammatory for disease states like arthritis, rheumatoid arthritis, and bursitis as well as inflammatory diseases of the gastrointestinal system, such as irritable bowel syndrome, food allergies, and leaky gut syndrome.

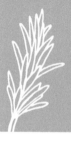

Azteca Hot Chocolate for Two

The three spices sacred to the Aztecs were cacao, cayenne, and vanilla; mixed together, they are a potent and delicious combination in this warming drink. I've added the silky texture of coconut milk and a creamy knob of Kerrygold Irish butter made from cows grazed exclusively on green grass. The raw cacao powder is rich in antioxidants and minerals that protect heart health.

GLUTEN-FREE, GRAIN-FREE, NUT-FREE, QUICK, VEGETARIAN

SERVES 2 | PREP TIME: 5 MINUTES | COOK TIME: 10 MINUTES

1 cup water

1 cup full-fat coconut milk

2 tablespoons unsalted Kerrygold Irish butter or any pastured butter (see tip)

1 tablespoon vanilla extract

1 tablespoon plus 1 teaspoon maple syrup

¼ cup raw cacao powder or high-quality, natural unsweetened cocoa powder

2 dashes cinnamon

Dash cayenne

1. In a small saucepan over medium-low heat, heat the water, coconut milk, butter, vanilla, and maple syrup until bubbles are forming at the edge of the pan.
2. In a mixing bowl, combine the cacao powder, cinnamon, and cayenne.
3. Remove the saucepan from the heat and slowly pour the hot milk into the mixing bowl.
4. Blend with an immersion blender or a whisk until frothy.
5. Divide the hot chocolate between 2 mugs and enjoy.

INGREDIENT TIP: Pastured butter is rich in fat-soluble vitamins A, D, and K₂ as well as CLA. CLA is an essential fatty acid found in grass-fed animals and may protect against heart disease, cancer, and type 2 diabetes.

CACAO/CHOCOLATE

Unprocessed cocoa, cacao powder, paste, nibs

SAFETY CONSIDERATIONS: None known

TASTE/ACTIVITY: BITTER/WARMING/DRYING

PROPERTIES: Antioxidant, hypotensive, mood elevator

USES: Supports heart health, lowers blood pressure and blood sugar levels

SUGGESTED PREPARATIONS: Candy, dessert, hot chocolate, infused honey or elixir; nibs mixed into granola or sprinkled on yogurt, smoothie

ESPECIALLY GOOD FOR: ANTIOXIDANTS

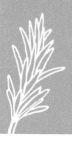

Cacao is a superfood that is extremely high in antioxidants, which protects cells from free radicals. It is high in minerals like magnesium, potassium, iron, chromium, and calcium. Cacao is beneficial to the heart and also lowers blood pressure and blood sugar levels. Cacao is also a great mood elevator.

Jalapeño Margarita

Herb-inspired cocktails are popular these days, and I admit that I also like to experiment with herbal cocktail combinations from time to time. Jalapeño margaritas at our local Mexican restaurant are a favorite date night treat, so of course, I had to develop my own version at home. I've found that the secret to a good jalapeño margarita is the addition of orange and cilantro muddled in the bottom of the shaker along with some cilantro and fresh jalapeño slices. Sour, sweet, pungent, and salty are all rolled up into one fancy beverage.

DAIRY-FREE, GLUTEN-FREE, GRAIN-FREE, NUT-FREE, QUICK, VEGAN

SERVES 2 | PREP TIME: 10 MINUTES

1 lime, quartered, divided

6 to 8 tablespoons sea salt or sugar

1 thick slice navel orange, plus 2 slices

½ jalapeño pepper, sliced, divided

8 cilantro sprigs, plus a few leaves
  for garnish

Crushed ice

4 ounces silver tequila

4 ounces freshly squeezed lime juice

2 ounces Cointreau orange liqueur

1. Rub two wedges of lime around the rim of two margarita glasses.
2. Fill a shallow saucer with the salt or sugar, then immediately dip the rims of the glasses in it.
3. Set the glasses aside while you mix the margarita.
4. Place the orange slice, the remaining 2 quarters of lime, half the jalapeño slices, and the cilantro in a cocktail shaker.
5. Muddle the ingredients with the back of a spoon to release their flavors.
6. Fill the shaker halfway with crushed ice.
7. Pour the tequila, lime juice, and Cointreau into the shaker.
8. Place the lid on tightly and shake until well chilled.
9. Strain the margarita from the shaker into the margarita glasses.
10. Garnish with the remaining jalapeño slices, orange slices, and a few leaves of fresh cilantro.

PREPARATION TIP: Choose 6 big juicy limes at the store. If you give your citrus a nice, firm roll on the counter before you halve them, you'll break up some of those little pulp pockets of juice and get more into your drink.

HERB PROFILE: See Cilantro (page 54).

Elderberry Hot Toddy Elixir

A classic hot toddy is best sipped when a chill has crept under your coat or you feel a cough or sore throat coming on. This potent elixir can be added to hot water and lemon for an instant hot toddy whenever you need it. In this recipe I've combined classic warming ingredients with elderberries for a value-added, antiviral pop. Be forewarned: The dried elderberries may abscond with some of your whiskey in the rehydration process. Make this elixir ahead of cold season and keep on hand through the winter.

DAIRY-FREE, GLUTEN-FREE, GRAIN-FREE, NUT-FREE, VEGETARIAN

MAKES 2 CUPS | PREP TIME: 5 MINUTES | COOK TIME: 1 HOUR, PLUS 1 HOUR TO STEEP

2 cups Irish whiskey

½ cup dried elderberries

2-inch knob fresh ginger, thinly sliced

1- to 3-inch cinnamon stick, broken

6 to 8 whole cloves

½ cup honey

1. Combine the whiskey, elderberries, ginger, cinnamon, and cloves in a medium saucepan.
2. Simmer for 1 hour on low heat, stirring occasionally. Do not boil.
3. Remove from the heat after 1 hour. Cover and allow to sit for 1 hour.
4. While the whiskey mixture is still warm, pour through a fine-mesh strainer into a mason jar. Discard the herbs and spices.
5. Clean the saucepan and return the whiskey to the pan.
6. Add the honey into the warm whiskey, and stir gently until well incorporated.
7. When completely cooled, decant into the mason jar or a nice liqueur bottle, and store in the pantry at room temperature.

SERVING TIP: To make a hot toddy, put 3 tablespoons elixir into the bottom of a mug, add a thick slice of lemon, and mash the lemon with the back of a spoon. Pour 1 cup of hot water into the mug and stir. Taste for sweetness. Add more honey (or elixir) if desired.

MAKE-AHEAD TIP: Make this hot toddy elixir well ahead of the cold and flu season this year and make some extra for gift giving over the holidays.

HERB PROFILE: See Elderberry (page 87), Ginger (page 49), and Cloves (page 115).

Lavender Lemonade

This is the quintessential herbal lemonade. While all lavenders have edible flowers, the English and Provence varieties are most often used for culinary purposes. Lavender is a sweet-smelling, but somewhat bitter-tasting, digestive carminative that also doubles as a relaxing nervine. Perfect to sip on a hot day with your feet up!

DAIRY-FREE, GLUTEN-FREE, GRAIN-FREE, NUT-FREE, VEGAN

SERVES 2 | PREP TIME: 20 MINUTES, PLUS 30 MINUTES TO INFUSE

¼ cup freshly picked lavender flowers, plus a few sprigs for garnish (or 1 tablespoon dried lavender flowers)

½ cup sugar, plus more if needed

1 cup boiling water

¾ cup freshly squeezed lemon juice, plus more if needed

1 cup or more cold water

Cracked ice

2 lemon slices

1. Place the lavender flowers in a large Pyrex or heatproof measuring bowl.
2. Pour the sugar over the flowers and gently rub the flowers into the sugar using the back of a spoon.
3. Pour the boiling water over the lavender sugar and stir until the sugar has dissolved.
4. Cover and let infuse for 30 minutes.
5. Strain the lavender-infused syrup and pour into a serving carafe or pitcher.
6. Stir in the lemon juice and cold water.
7. Taste and adjust for tartness or sweetness by adding more lemon juice or sugar. Add the cracked ice.
8. Add the lemon slices and a few lavender sprigs to the serving pitcher and serve immediately.

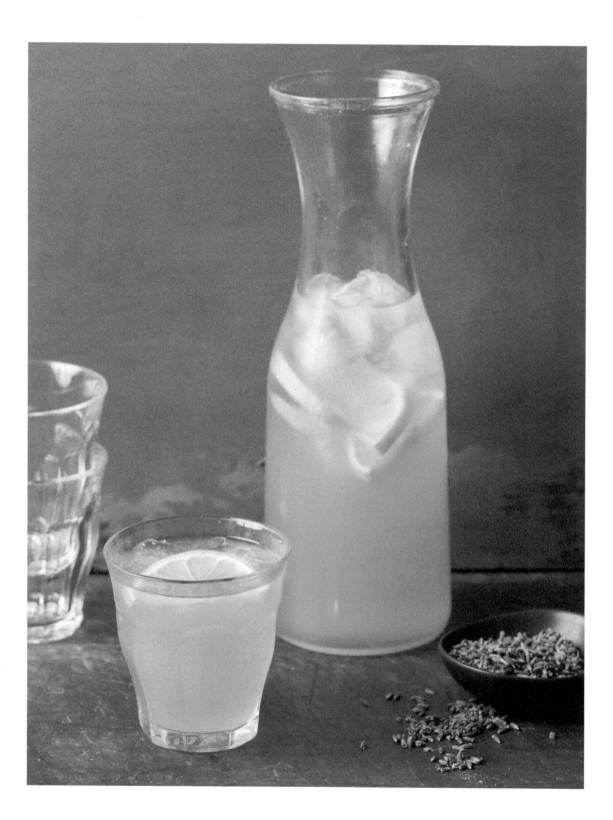

LAVENDER

Fresh or dried flower buds

SAFETY CONSIDERATIONS: None known

TASTE/ACTIVITY: BITTER/AROMATIC/COOL/DRY

PROPERTIES: Anodyne, antiseptic, antispasmodic, antiviral, carminative mild antidepressant, relaxing nervine

USES: Relieves digestive spasms, gas, bloating, and nausea; treats intestinal viruses and bacteria to the bowel

SUGGESTED PREPARATIONS: Baking, infused honey, infused syrup, tea

ESPECIALLY GOOD FOR: CALMING

Lavender is a mild antidepressant and relaxing nervine that helps calm the nervous system in times of stress or tension.

Peach Ginger Shrub

A fruit shrub is a sweetened vinegar drink popular during the colonial era, when an abundance of overripe fruit was preserved by simmering in equal parts vinegar and sugar, molasses, or honey. Fruit shrubs have made a comeback and are now affectionately called "drinking vinegars." Cherries, blackberries, blueberries, peaches, elderberries, cranberries, and even fresh ginger make exceptionally good shrubs. If you have difficulty drinking 8 glasses of water daily, adding a splash of vinegar-based fruit shrubs will make it that much easier. You'll also be getting a nice boost of vitamins, minerals, and antioxidants in every sip.

DAIRY-FREE, GLUTEN-FREE, GRAIN-FREE, NUT-FREE, VEGETARIAN

**MAKES 2 CUPS | PREP TIME: 20 MINUTES
COOK TIME: 30 MINUTES, PLUS 12 TO 24 HOURS TO INFUSE**

1 cup raw apple cider vinegar

1 cup honey

2 cups sliced ripe peaches

¼ cup chopped fresh ginger, or 1 tablespoon plus 1 teaspoon ground ginger

1. In a medium saucepan, heat the vinegar and honey together on low heat to create a syrupy mixture.
2. Add the peach slices and ginger, and simmer until the fruit collapses and the ginger becomes fragrant, about 30 minutes. Do not boil.
3. Cover, turn off the heat, and allow to infuse overnight.
4. The next day, strain the finished shrub into a clean pint-size, wide-mouth mason jar. Cover, label, and store in the refrigerator.

TO USE: Shrubs are incredibly versatile. To use a fruit shrub in a drink, put 1 to 3 tablespoons into a mug of hot water for "tea," or over ice with sparkling water. Use this sweet/sour vinegar in salad dressings or meat marinades by adding olive oil.

SUBSTITUTION TIP: This recipe is wonderful for experimenting with different flavors. A few more suggested combinations: elderberries and warming spices, blackberries and sage leaf, rhubarb and hibiscus flowers, blueberries and lemon verbena, and prickly pear cactus fruit and basil.

HERB PROFILE: See Ginger (page 49).

Aromatic Chai Tea Blend

The secret to a great cup of exotic carminative-charged chai is to lightly toast whole spices in the oven first. Breaking open the toasted spices with a rap of a rolling pin will release their pungent aroma so that the hot water can receive it. Just a few tablespoons of mixed spices and a few minutes of prep will give you enough aromatic tea blend to make about 16 cups. This tea is the perfect start to your day or to serve after a big meal to help digest it.

DAIRY-FREE, GLUTEN-FREE, GRAIN-FREE, NUT-FREE, QUICK, VEGETARIAN

MAKES 1 CUP OF DRY TEA BLEND | PREP TIME: 15 MINUTES | COOK TIME: 15 MINUTES

2 tablespoons broken cinnamon sticks

1 tablespoon chopped fresh ginger

1 tablespoon fennel seeds

2 teaspoons ground cardamom

1 teaspoon whole cloves

½ teaspoon whole black peppercorns

½ teaspoon coriander

½ cup loose black tea leaves

1. Preheat the oven to 350°F.
2. Place the cinnamon, ginger, fennel, cardamom, cloves, peppercorns, and coriander on a baking sheet. Toast for 5 minutes or until the spices are aromatic. Let cool on the stovetop.
3. Crush the spices lightly by covering them with a paper bag and then rolling over the bag with a rolling pin.
4. In a bowl, toss the spices and black tea together until well blended.
5. Store in a glass jar with a tight-fitting lid.

FOR 1 CUP OF CHAI TEA

1 cup water

1 tablespoon Aromatic Chai Tea Blend

½ cup full-fat coconut milk

Honey

Bring the water to a boil in a small saucepan and add the chai tea blend. Cover to keep the aromatic oils in the tea. Reduce the heat to low and simmer for 15 minutes. Remove from the heat and let steep for about 10 minutes. Add the milk; reheat until hot. Strain out the spices using a small fine-mesh strainer and sweeten with honey to taste.

INGREDIENT TIP: Traditionally, black tea is always a part of this recipe, but if you are averse to caffeine, you can leave it out and simply use the spice blend all by itself.

HERB PROFILE: See Cinnamon (page 35), Ginger (page 49), Fennel (page 77), and Cardamom (page 39).

Rose Lassi

A lassi is a traditional frothy Indian yogurt drink. In this recipe, the rose and yogurt are both sweet and cooling, reducing heat and inflammation (useful if you've been eating hot and spicy curry dishes). The most commonly known lassi by far is the mango lassi, which is readily available on the menu in most Indian restaurants. But rose lassi is appropriate for a special meal, say, on Valentine's Day, or simply when you need to give yourself a rose petal hug.

GLUTEN-FREE, GRAIN-FREE, QUICK, VEGETARIAN

SERVES 1 | PREP TIME: 10 MINUTES

1 cup yogurt

1/4 cup cold milk

1 tablespoon rose petal syrup (made from the Basic Herb-Infused Syrup recipe on page 133) or Rose Petal Jam (page 47)

1½ teaspoons sugar

¼ teaspoon ground cardamom

6 ice cubes

1 tablespoon combined finely chopped almonds, pistachios, and rose petals (optional)

1. Put the yogurt and milk in a blender.
2. Add the rose syrup, sugar, cardamom, and ice cubes, and blend well until frothy.
3. Pour the lassi into a tall serving glass.
4. Garnish with the chopped almonds, pistachios, and rose petals, if desired.
5. Serve immediately.

SUBSTITUTION TIP: If you don't have access to fresh fragrant rose petals, there are sources to purchase good-quality ready-made rose syrup and jam online (see Resources, page 185). Royal Rose brand Rose Simple Syrup and Rose Petal Spread made by Maharishi Ayurveda are two good options. Both products are certified organic and contain no artificial colors or flavors. They are well worth the price and will last years in your refrigerator after opening.

ROSE

Dried rose hips, fresh or dried flowers (unsprayed or certified organic)

SAFETY CONSIDERATIONS: Allergies to roses

TASTE/ACTIVITY: SWEET/ASTRINGENT/COOL/DRY (petals); SOUR (hips)

PROPERTIES: Antidepressant, anti-inflammatory, astringent, relaxant nervine, tonic to the heart and female reproductive system

USES: Supports heart health; soothes broken heart, grief, heartache, loss, inflammation in the body, too much time in the sun, and fever

SUGGESTED PREPARATIONS: Tea, jam, infused syrup, infused vinegar, and infused oxymel

ESPECIALLY GOOD FOR: CALMING

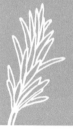

Rose petals are considered a heart-settling nervine and tonic for the heart. Relaxing nervines help calm the nervous system in times of stress and tension. Rose is used in Chinese, Ayurvedic, and Western herbal traditions as an antidepressant and treatment for grief and heartache. It is also used to "open" an emotionally closed, wounded, or shut-down heart.

Sage Oxymel

An oxymel (from Latin, meaning "acid and honey") combines equal parts vinegar and honey, warmed thoroughly over low heat to create a syrupy mixture, to which herbs and spices are added. Vinegar is a wonderful medium for extracting beneficial compounds, minerals, and aromatic flavors. In this case, sage provides antiviral, antibacterial, anti-inflammatory, and drying activity, the perfect combination for a sore throat or a runny nose.

DAIRY-FREE, GLUTEN-FREE, GRAIN-FREE, NUT-FREE, VEGETARIAN

**MAKES 2 CUPS | PREP TIME: 20 MINUTES
COOK TIME: 30 MINUTES, PLUS 12 TO 24 HOURS TO INFUSE**

1 cup raw apple cider vinegar

1 cup honey

2 cups fresh sage or 1 cup dried sage

1. Place the vinegar and honey together in a medium saucepan and heat just enough to create a syrupy mixture. Do not boil.
2. Add the sage and heat through just until it becomes fragrant. Cover and turn off the heat, and allow the oxymel to infuse overnight.
3. The next morning, strain the oxymel into a pint-size, wide-mouth mason jar. Cover, label, and store in the pantry at room temperature.

TO USE: Add 1 to 3 tablespoons of oxymel into a mug of hot water for "tea" or into a glass of fizzy water with cracked ice, or use in salad dressings or marinades for meats by adding to olive oil.

SUBSTITUTION TIP: Rose petals, bee balm, thyme, and lemon balm all make delicious oxymels if you'd like to experiment with other tastes.

HERB PROFILE: See Sage (page 111).

Still Room Amaro

A few years ago, I was exploring a local spirits store, where some beautiful amaro bottles caught my eye. *Amaro* is the Italian word for "bitter," and Italy is famous for its wide variety of bitter-sweet aperitifs. I've always crafted my own digestive bitters using dandelion root, citrus peel, and warming spices, but that was the first time I purchased an Italian version with many of the same ingredients. I've tweaked my old tried-and-true recipe here to embrace the Italian tradition. Initially, the bitter taste of dandelion root may be a challenging one to embrace, but I urge you to continue while your taste buds become accustomed to this unfamiliar sensation! The physical rewards of improved digestion will benefit you from the inside out.

DAIRY-FREE, GLUTEN-FREE, GRAIN-FREE, NUT-FREE, VEGAN

MAKES 3 CUPS | PREP TIME: 15 MINUTES, PLUS 6 WEEKS TO INFUSE

1 teaspoon dried chamomile flowers

1 teaspoon dried fennel seeds

3 whole cloves

2 tablespoons toasted walnuts

1 orange, preferably organic

1 tablespoon dried dandelion root

1 tablespoon minced fresh mint

1 tablespoon minced fresh rosemary

1 tablespoon minced fresh sage

1 vanilla bean

½ teaspoon coriander

3 cups vodka or Everclear (100 to 150 proof is best to extract the resins and bitter compounds)

1 cup water

1 cup sugar

1. Place the chamomile, fennel seeds, cloves, and toasted walnuts in a paper bag and rap with a rolling pin a few times to them. Put the cracked spices and nuts in a quart-size mason jar.
2. Using a vegetable peeler, remove the zest from the orange (no white pith) and cut zest into thin strips.
3. Add the orange zest, dandelion root, mint, rosemary, sage, and vanilla bean to the jar.
4. Add the vodka or Everclear. Stir, cover, and label with the contents and date. Allow to infuse in a dark place for 6 weeks. Mark 6 weeks ahead on your calendar so you don't forget to strain it.

〉〉〉〉〉〉

5. After 6 weeks, strain the liquid through a fine-mesh strainer into a clean 1-quart mason jar. Discard the solids.
6. Make a simple syrup by warming the water and sugar together over medium heat until the sugar has dissolved.
7. Add the warm syrup (or substitute honey or maple syrup) by ¼-cup increments to the herb-infused vodka, stirring thoroughly and tasting as you go until you get the right combination of bitter and sweet for your taste.
8. The amaro will mellow and taste better and better with age.

TO USE: Sip ½ to 1 ounce while preparing a meal to stimulate digestion and increase nutrient absorption up to 3 times per day. It's best to use your bitter elixir 15 to 30 minutes before meals.

DANDELION ROOT

Dried root

SAFETY CONSIDERATIONS: None known

TASTE/ACTIVITY: BITTER/SLIGHTLY SWEET/COOL/MOIST

PROPERTIES: Alterative, cholagogue, hepatoprotective, mild diuretic, mild laxative, nutritive tonic

USES: Aids digestion and proper absorption of nutrients; treats sluggish bowel, chronic constipation, and liver distress from fatty foods, environmental toxins, drug and alcohol use, and chemotherapy

SUGGESTED PREPARATIONS: Bitters tincture, tea

ESPECIALLY GOOD FOR: LIVER HEALTH

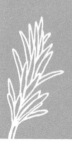

One of the best liver herbs, dandelion root stimulates bile secretions, small intestine enzymes, and pancreatic enzymes, which are essential for digestion and nutrient absorption. It stimulates the growth of healthy bowel flora; decreases liver distress from fatty foods, drug or alcohol abuse, gallstones, and chemotherapy; helps liver and kidneys improve elimination; may improve acne and eczema-like skin conditions; and regulates hormone balance. It is very safe for children (and adults) with constipation.

CHAPTER NINE

SWEET TREATS

I am often reminded that the sweet taste, in moderation, is indeed a nourishing one, and that some of the finest and most medicinal herbs and spices can be incorporated into desserts. Sweet treats lend themselves perfectly to after-dinner carminatives, such as warming ginger, cinnamon, lavender, and thyme.

Lavender Pistachio Biscotti

Twenty years ago, I began experimenting with adding herbs and spices to my basic biscotti recipe, and I've shared hundreds of them with friends and family over the years. This aromatic lavender-infused biscotti is certainly a big favorite. Lavender is a relaxing nervine (it calms the nerves) and carminative (digestive aid) that pairs beautifully with chamomile tea after dinner, or any time.

VEGETARIAN

MAKES 14 BISCOTTI | PREP TIME: 15 MINUTES, PLUS 30 MINUTES TO COOL
COOK TIME: 55 MINUTES

½ cup shelled pistachio nuts

8 tablespoons (1 stick) unsalted butter,
   at room temperature

¾ cups sugar

1 tablespoon dried lavender flower buds

1 teaspoon vanilla extract

2 eggs

2 cups unbleached flour,
   plus more for kneading

1½ teaspoons baking powder

½ teaspoon salt

1. Preheat the oven to 325°F.
2. Toast the pistachios in a pan over medium heat, shaking constantly until slightly brown, about 5 minutes. When cool, roughly chop and set aside.
3. In a mixing bowl, cream the butter and sugar with a hand mixer until well blended.
4. Add the lavender buds, vanilla, and eggs, and beat until frothy.
5. In a large bowl, combine the flour, baking powder, and salt. Stir to combine well.
6. Add the dry ingredients to the creamed mixture and continue beating until well combined. Fold in the nuts.
7. With floured hands, remove the cookie batter from the bowl. It will be fairly wet and sticky.
8. Sprinkle a bit of flour on the countertop and knead it into cookie dough until it is manageable. Don't overwork the dough.
9. Form a long cookie log 3 inches wide and 12 to 14 inches long. Smooth out any cracks or holes. Place on a baking sheet.

10. Bake the cookie log for 25 to 30 minutes. It should still show a finger indentation when pressed.
11. Let it cool for 30 minutes. Using a serrated knife, cut the biscotti into 1-inch-thick slices.
12. Spread out the biscotti on the same baking sheet and bake for an additional 15 to 20 minutes. Allow to cool completely.
13. The biscotti should be very crispy. Store in an airtight container.

SUBSTITUTION TIP: I have successfully swapped out the 1 tablespoon of lavender flower buds with an equal amount of anise seeds or chopped crystallized ginger. You can also swap out the pistachios for chopped almonds or hazelnuts.

HERB PROFILE: See Lavender (page 154).

Crystallized Ginger Candy

Ginger candy is a versatile culinary ingredient that can add a pungent surprise when chopped and stirred into cookie batter, gingerbread, fruit salads, or baked apples. It's also a great travel companion to help ease motion sickness, nausea, and digestive spasms while on the road. You will need a candy thermometer for this recipe.

DAIRY-FREE, GLUTEN-FREE, GRAIN-FREE, NUT-FREE, VEGAN

MAKES 12 OUNCES | PREP TIME: 10 MINUTES
COOK TIME: 30 MINUTES, PLUS 1 HOUR TO SOAK AND 24 TO 48 HOURS TO DRY

1 pound fresh ginger

4 cups sugar, plus more for coating the ginger slices

4 cups water

Pinch salt

1. Peel the ginger with a sharp paring knife.
2. Cut the ginger into ⅛-inch-thick uniform slices.
3. Combine the sugar and water in a deep stainless-steel pot. Heat over medium heat and stir continuously until the sugar has dissolved.
4. Add the salt and the ginger slices. Simmer for about 20 minutes and then increase the heat until the syrup reaches 225°F. (This is where you'll need the candy thermometer.)
5. Remove from the heat. Cover and let the ginger sit in the syrup for a minimum of 1 hour or overnight.

6. To coat the ginger slices with sugar, warm the ginger and syrup again until the syrup thins. When they are hot, lift the ginger pieces out of the syrup with a slotted spoon or tongs, allowing excess syrup to drip back into the pot, and transfer to a wide tray.

7. Toss the warm ginger slices with sugar to coat. Shake off any excess sugar, and spread the coated ginger slices out on a cooling rack for a day or two, until they are dry.

8. The crystallized ginger can be stored in a covered container at room temperature for a few months or up to a year.

INGREDIENT TIP: The ginger syrup and ginger sugar created in the making of this recipe can be repurposed. Simply put the ginger syrup in a clean mason jar, label it, and store in the refrigerator for up to 1 month. You can make a quick ginger ale by adding 2 tablespoons syrup to a glass of sparkling water or make a hot ginger tea by adding it to a mug of hot water. The ginger sugar can be stored in a jar in your pantry at room temperature. Use it to make gingerbread cookies or pumpkin pie.

HERB PROFILE: See Ginger (page 49).

Poached Pears with Elderberry and Warming Spices

Poached pears make a simple, elegant dessert that takes only a few minutes of prep. The rest of the time is spent allowing the pears to slowly absorb the fragrant poaching liquid and then to chill. These red jewels are well worth the wait. Any use of elderberry preparations during the fall and winter months can be a boon to keeping the immune system on guard. But you'll enjoy this dessert mostly because it tastes so good.

GLUTEN-FREE, GRAIN-FREE, NUT-FREE, VEGAN

SERVES 4 | PREP TIME: 20 MINUTES, PLUS 4 HOURS TO CHILL | COOK TIME: 40 MINUTES

1½ cups elderberry shrub (see page 155)

1½ cups dry red wine

½ cup sugar (or substitute maple syrup)

1 (1-by-4-inch) strip orange peel

2 cinnamon sticks, broken into pieces

3 whole cloves

4 firm Red Anjou or Bosc pears

1. Combine the elderberry shrub, red wine, sugar, orange peel, cinnamon sticks, and cloves in a large saucepan. Bring to a boil until the sugar dissolves. Reduce the heat to medium-low.
2. While the poaching liquid is simmering, peel the pears with a vegetable peeler, leaving the stem intact. Create a flat bottom on each pear by slicing off just enough so that the pears can stand upright at serving time.
3. Place the pears on their sides in the poaching liquid. Reduce the heat to low and simmer for 20 minutes. Gently turn them every 5 minutes with a spoon to ensure even color. The pears should be cooked but still firm. Remove the pan from the heat and cool to room temperature, turning the pears occasionally.
4. When the pears have cooled, cover and refrigerate them in the poaching liquid for at least 4 hours, but no more than 24 hours, turning occasionally.
5. To serve, carefully remove the pears from the poaching liquid and place upright on individual serving plates.

6. Strain the poaching liquid and return it to the saucepan. Bring to a boil, then reduce heat and cook until reduced by half, about 20 minutes. The liquid should be slightly thickened and syrupy.
7. Let the syrup cool to warm. Drizzle the pears with the syrup. Serve with a small scoop of vanilla ice cream, if desired.

PREPARATION TIP: This dessert needs to be planned a day or two ahead to allow the pears to soak in the garnet-colored liquid. It's worth the extra planning; these make an impressive presentation.

HERB PROFILE: See Elderberry (page 87).

Lavender Ganache Truffles

Who doesn't love a small but decadent nibble of chocolate? Who doesn't relish it even more with the essence of herbs and spices infused into it? The shining nutritional star in this recipe is the chocolate, of course. While cacao and cocoa come from the exact same plant, cocoa is highly processed. Without processing, cacao retains its incredibly high level of antioxidant power. Cacao also has a wealth of vitamins and minerals, including calcium, magnesium, iron, and potassium.

GLUTEN-FREE, GRAIN-FREE, NUT-FREE, VEGETARIAN

**MAKES 30 TRUFFLES | PREP TIME: 5 MINUTES
COOK TIME: 15 MINUTES, PLUS 15 MINUTES TO INFUSE AND 2 HOURS TO CHILL**

1 cup heavy whipping cream

2 tablespoons unsalted butter

2 tablespoons honey

⅓ cup dried lavender flower buds

2 (3-ounce) high-quality 72 percent cacao chocolate bars, finely chopped

2 ounces unprocessed raw cacao powder or high-quality, natural unsweetened cocoa powder, plus more for rolling the truffles

1. Place the cream, butter, and honey in a double boiler. Heat over medium heat until you see steam rising and small bubbles forming around the edge but the mixture is not quite boiling. Stir in the lavender, cover, and turn off the heat. Allow the lavender to infuse in the cream for 15 minutes.

2. Place the chocolate and the cacao powder into a large mixing bowl. When the lavender cream is infused, strain it through a fine-mesh sieve directly into the bowl of chocolate. Allow to stand for 2 minutes to melt the chocolate.

3. After 2 minutes, whisk the mixture until it is smooth and shiny. A stick blender works well here but is not necessary.

4. Cover the bowl. Put the bowl and 2 teaspoons in the refrigerator to chill for 2 to 5 hours. Do not freeze.

5. Place the cacao powder for rolling in a shallow pan. Line a baking sheet with parchment paper.

6. Ready to roll? Warm hands make truffle-rolling a challenge, so be sure to run your hands under very cold water (then dry them) or hold a gel ice pack or a bag of frozen veggies. Cold, dry hands will allow you to roll the truffles successfully.

7. Scoop a teaspoonful of chocolate and form into a ball between your hands, working quickly. Dip the ball into the cacao powder and place on the prepared baking sheet. Repeat. You may need to chill your hands multiple times.

8. Refrigerate the finished truffles in a sealed container. They should last for a few weeks (with expert discipline!).

SUBSTITUTION TIP: Lavender is just one herb you can have fun with in this recipe. Imagine swapping out the lavender for pungent ginger, fragrant rose petals, or a few teaspoons of instant espresso powder, cardamom, or orange zest. Whatever flavor you choose, these make great holiday gifts. You might even want to buy fancy foil candy cups and boxes (available at most craft stores) to present them in.

HERB PROFILE: See Cacao/Chocolate (page 149).

Herbal Tea Frozen Popsicles

Making your own popsicles instead of buying artificially colored, high-fructose-corn-syrup varieties is fast and healthier. Popsicle molds are readily found online or in the seasonal summer section of your grocery store. Nothing lights up a child's face faster than a refreshing peppermint popsicle on a hot day, or a ginger or chamomile popsicle when they are feeling sick or grumpy. Herbal tea popsicles aren't just for children, either. You can experiment with any flavor tea you're fond of, or even add sliced fruit if so inclined. The only hard part of making these tasty treats is waiting for them to freeze.

DAIRY-FREE, GLUTEN-FREE, GRAIN-FREE, NUT-FREE, VEGETARIAN

MAKES 10 POPSICLES
PREP TIME: 5 MINUTES, PLUS 10 MINUTES TO STEEP AND 4 HOURS TO FREEZE

5 tea bags (such as peppermint, chamomile, or ginger)

4 cups boiling water

4 teaspoons freshly squeezed lemon juice

4 to 6 teaspoons honey

1. Put the tea bags in the mason jar, and cover with boiling water up to the shoulder of the jar.
2. Allow the tea to steep for 10 minutes.
3. Discard the tea bags.
4. Stir in the lemon juice and honey with a wooden spoon until the honey is dissolved. Cool to room temperature.
5. Pour the sweetened tea into popsicle molds and freeze until solid, 4 hours or more.

PREPARATION TIP: If you don't have a popsicle mold, don't be discouraged. When I was small, we made popsicles in small plastic cups with wooden popsicle sticks. Old school isn't so bad. They both work equally well.

HERB PROFILE: See Mint (page 73), Chamomile (page 176), and Ginger (page 49).

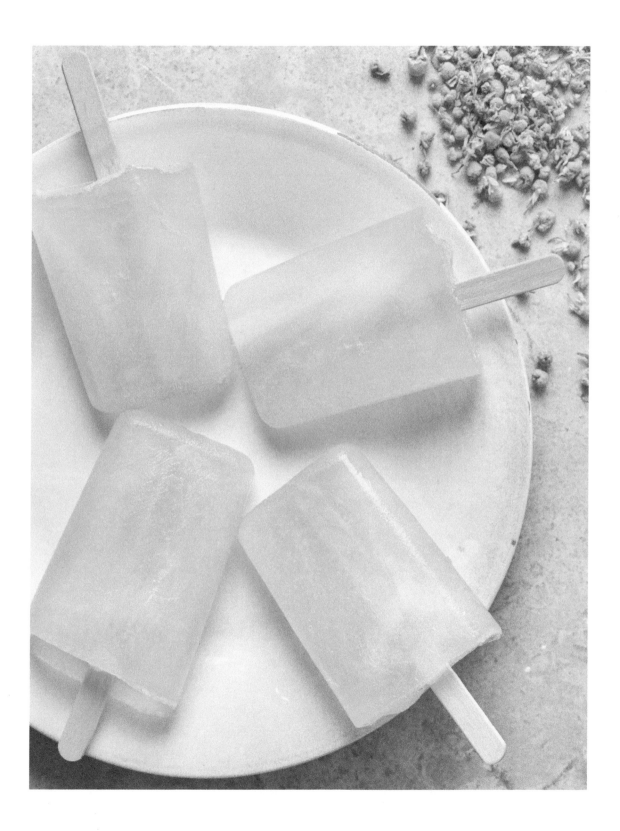

CHAMOMILE

Fresh or dried flowers

SAFETY CONSIDERATIONS: None known

TASTE/ACTIVITY: SWEET/SLIGHTLY BITTER/WARM/MOIST

PROPERTIES: Anti-inflammatory, antispasmodic, carminative, mild sedative

USES: In children, alleviates irritability, nightmares, growing pains, colic, bellyaches, and teeth-grinding or teething. In adults, treats anxiety or stress symptoms centralized to the stomach, irritable bowel syndrome, diverticulitis, stress induced ulcers, excess gastric acid, cramps, colds and flu, hyperactivity, attention-deficit hyperactivity disorder, headaches, nausea, vomiting, menstrual cramps, premenstrual anxiety and irritability, mood swings, mild insomnia, muscle cramps, and back spasms.

SUGGESTED PREPARATIONS: Frozen tea ice pops, infused syrup, infused tea

ESPECIALLY GOOD FOR: STRESS RELIEF

Chamomile combats worry or stress internalized to the digestive system that results in nervous tummy or digestive upset.

Honeyed Gorgonzola Stuffed Figs with Thyme

Fruit and cheese make a fine end to any meal. The addition of honey and fresh thyme turns this simple dish into an elegant dessert. When our fig tree is laden with ripe fruit, I can't think of a better way to celebrate the abundance. The volatile oils in thyme are a potent remedy for infections, particularly in the respiratory and digestive tracts. Served with crisp white wine, this dessert could easily become a light dinner.

GLUTEN-FREE, GRAIN-FREE, QUICK, VEGETARIAN

SERVES 4 | PREP TIME: 10 MINUTES | COOK TIME: 5 MINUTES

8 medium figs

3 ounces gorgonzola cheese

2 tablespoons walnuts, finely chopped

2 tablespoons chopped fresh thyme

¼ cup honey

1. Preheat the oven 375°F.
2. Remove the fig stems and cut a deep X in the top of each fig.
3. Gently open the top of each fig with the tip of a teaspoon and stuff with about 1 heaping teaspoon of the gorgonzola.
4. Sprinkle the stuffed figs with the nuts and fresh thyme. Place in a baking dish.
5. Drizzle with the honey.
6. Bake for about 5 minutes, or until the figs look soft and release some juice.
7. Serve warm.

SUBSTITUTION TIP: You may substitute ricotta or goat cheese if you aren't fond of gorgonzola's strong flavor.

HERB PROFILE: See Thyme (page 97).

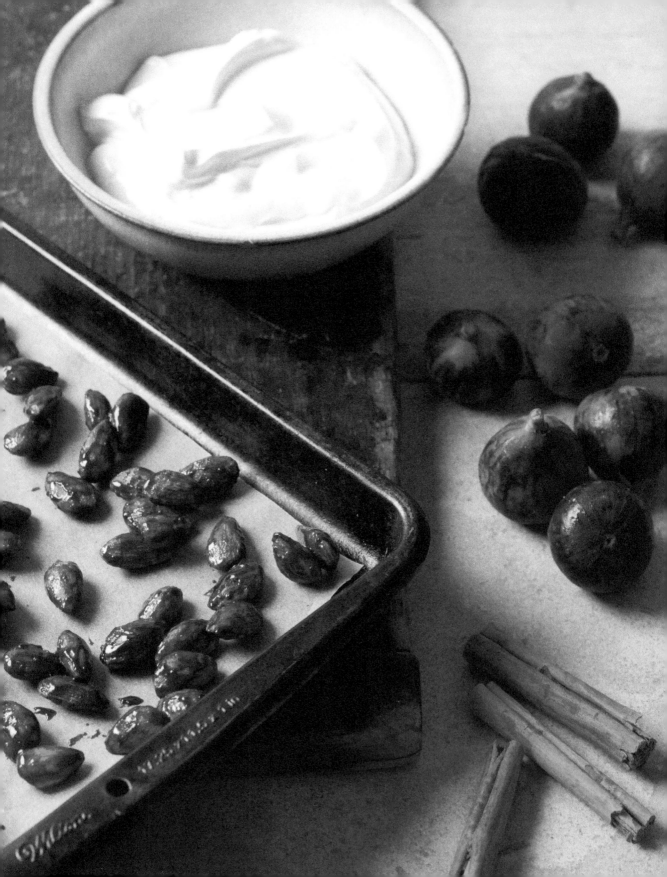

Appendix:
ENERGETICS OF COMMON AILMENTS

The medicinal use of culinary herbs can help you heal from common ailments like coughs, cold, flu, or digestive upset. By choosing the right herbs, you can ease uncomfortable symptoms such as a stuffy nose, productive cough, gas, bloating, or indigestion. We've included this appendix to provide some general examples of how the energetics of symptoms can be observed and how the energetics of culinary herbs can be utilized to help a few acute conditions.

COLD/DAMP Symptoms

*respond well to warming/drying herbs

- » chills; uncomfortable in cold weather; need to "bundle up"
- » acute onset of cold/flu virus
- » profuse mucus, clear, or opaque in color
- » productive wet cough
- » belching, gas, flatulence, poor digestion

Remember, the pungent/spicy taste is generally warming and drying, and characterizes a wide variety of common culinary herbs such as garlic, ginger, thyme, oregano, cinnamon, and horseradish, just to name a few. Pungent/spicy herbs are also antiviral, antibacterial, carminative and expectorating. Herbs and foods with the sour taste, such as lemons, elderberries, and vinegar are also drying and help tonify boggy mucus membranes, and many provide extra Vitamin C. The sour taste also stimulates the liver and gall bladder to help improve the digestive process.

HOT/DRY Symptoms

*respond well to cooling/moistening herbs

- » red, inflamed mucus membranes
- » dry, difficult to expectorate mucus; often yellow or green in color
- » unproductive cough

Unfortunately, there are very few cooling/moistening herbs used in a culinary setting. However, you may be able to utilize some of the pungent-tasting herbs—such onions, garlic, horseradish, and ginger (see page 132)—to stimulate circulation and help fight off viral infections.

To study the energetics and symptoms of herbs, as well as overall energetic constitution of people, more deeply, please explore Rosalee de la Forêt's website (www.HerbswithRosalee.com) and her book *Alchemy of Herbs*. Rosalee also offers a free online mini course about herbal energetics that explores a wide and expansive variety of medicinal herbs, including some culinary ones.

THE DIRTY DOZEN™ & THE CLEAN FIFTEEN™

A nonprofit environmental watchdog organization called Environmental Working Group looks at data supplied by the U.S. Department of Agriculture and the Food and Drug Administration about pesticide residues. Each year it compiles a list of the best and worst pesticide loads found in commercial crops. You can use these lists to decide which fruits and vegetables to buy organic to minimize your exposure to pesticides and which produce is considered safe enough to buy conventionally. This does not mean they are pesticide-free, though, so wash these fruits and vegetables thoroughly.

The Dirty Dozen™

apples	nectarines	spinach
celery	peaches	strawberries
cherries	pears	sweet bell peppers
grapes	potatoes	tomatoes

Additionally, nearly three-quarters of hot pepper samples contained pesticide residues.

The Clean Fifteen™

asparagus	cauliflower	onions
avocados	eggplants	papayas
broccoli	honeydew melons	pineapples
cabbages	kiwis	sweet corn
cantaloupes	mangos	sweet peas (frozen)

MEASUREMENT CONVERSIONS

VOLUME EQUIVALENTS (LIQUID)

STANDARD	U.S. STANDARD (OUNCES)	METRIC (APPROXIMATE)
2 tablespoons	1 fl. oz.	30 mL
¼ cup	2 fl. oz.	60 mL
½ cup	4 fl. oz.	120 mL
1 cup	8 fl. oz.	240 mL
1½ cups	12 fl. oz.	355 mL
2 cups or 1 pint	16 fl. oz.	475 mL
4 cups or 1 quart	32 fl. oz.	1 L
1 gallon	128 fl. oz.	4 L

OVEN TEMPERATURES

FAHRENHEIT (F)	CELSIUS (C) (APPROXIMATE)
250°	120°
300°	150°
325°	165°
350°	180°
375°	190°
400°	200°
425°	220°
450°	230°

VOLUME EQUIVALENTS (DRY)

STANDARD	METRIC (APPROXIMATE)
⅛ teaspoon	0.5 mL
¼ teaspoon	1 mL
½ teaspoon	2 mL
¾ teaspoon	4 mL
1 teaspoon	5 mL
1 tablespoon	15 mL
¼ cup	59 mL
⅓ cup	79 mL
½ cup	118 mL
⅔ cup	156 mL
¾ cup	177 mL
1 cup	235 mL
2 cups or 1 pint	475 mL
3 cups	700 mL
4 cups or 1 quart	1 L

WEIGHT EQUIVALENTS

STANDARD	METRIC (APPROXIMATE)
½ ounce	15 g
1 ounce	30 g
2 ounces	60 g
4 ounces	115 g
8 ounces	225 g
12 ounces	340 g
16 ounces or 1 pound	455 g

GLOSSARY

ACUTE: Has the property of an illness or condition of sudden onset, such as fever or a viral or bacterial infection

ADAPTOGEN: An herb that increases the body's ability to resist the damaging effects of stress and restores normal physiological function

ALTERATIVE: Herbs that help support and restore balance and function to the bowel, liver, kidneys and skin. Sometimes called cleansing herbs

ANODYNE: Helps reduce and soothe pain

ANTIBACTERIAL: Helps prevent the growth of bacteria and resists pathogenic microorganisms

ANTIOXIDANT: Substance found in fruits, vegetables, and herbs that may prevent or delay some types of cell damage that lead to degenerative diseases

ANTIMICROBIAL: Kills and inhibits the growth of microorganisms

ANTISEPTIC: Reduces the possibility of infection

ANTISPASMODIC: Reduces cramping, muscle spasms, and spasmodic pains

ANTIVIRAL: Fights viral infections

BITTER: Serves as a stimulant to aid digestion beginning with the taste buds, promotes the proper breakdown of foods, assists in nutrient absorption and regular elimination

BIOAVAILABILITY: The extent to which nutrients are made more readily available for absorption/systemic circulation

BRONCHODILATOR: Helps to open and expand the airways in the lungs

CARMINATIVE: Contains volatile oils that help prevent gas from forming and assists in expelling it

CHELATE: To bind and remove heavy metals from the bloodstream

CHOLAGOGUE: Stimulates the flow of bile from the liver and gall bladder

CHRONIC: Persistent or long-lasting or a disease that comes slowly with time

DEMULCENT: Has mucilaginous qualities that are soothing to irritated or inflamed internal tissues

DIAPHORETIC: Helps promote perspiration

DIURETIC: Promotes the production and secretion of urine

EMMENAGOGUE: Helps stimulate menstruation

EXPECTORANT: Helps expel excess mucus from the system

FLAVONOIDS: Beneficial plant chemicals in fruits, vegetables, and herbs that are associated with prevention of cancer and cardiovascular and neurodegenerative diseases

GALACTAGOGUE: Helps increase the production of a mother's breast milk

HEPATOPROTECTIVE: An herb that has the ability to prevent damage to the liver

HOMEOSTASIS: The ability of the internal workings of the body to stay balanced and stable, regardless of external influences and conditions

HYPOTENSIVE: Lowers blood pressure

IMMUNE AMPHOTERIC: Helps regulate and balance the immune system, whether it is hyperfunctioning (in the case of allergies) or severely depleted (in the case of cancer)

LAXATIVE: Promotes bowel movement

MASTITIS: Breast infection generally related to breastfeeding

NERVINE: Calms and soothes the nerves and reduces tension and anxiety

NUTRITIVE: Nourishes and builds bodily tissues

SEDATIVE: Hase a soothing or calming effect on the body, thereby relieving anxiety, insomnia, and stress

STIMULANT: Increases metabolic activity and energy in the body

TONIC: Acts slowly and steadily to restore and strengthen an entire system, producing and restoring normal tone; generally taken over an extended period of time

RESOURCES

David Winston's Center for Herbal Studies I received formal training with my mentor, David Winston, RH (AHG), starting in 1994. Currently David offers on-site (New Jersey) and online educational opportunities for those who want to go deeper. David is an herbalist and ethnobotanist with over 40 years of training in Cherokee, Chinese, and Western herbal traditions. He is the founder/director of the Herbal Therapeutics Research Library and the dean of David Winston's Center for Herbal Studies, a two-year training program in clinical herbal medicine. www.HerbalTherapeutics.net

The Essential Herbal This magazine has been part of my welcome packet for new students since the very beginning. One of the original publications about herbs, *The Essential Herbal* is a bi-monthly print magazine that showcases articles from a wide range of herbalists, including its founding editor (and coauthor of this book), Tina Sams. www.EssentialHerbal.com

American Herbalist Guild The American Herbalists Guild has been in existence since 1989. An educational organization that hosts a yearly conference as well as listings for herbal schools and programs around the country, regional chapters and a directory of registered practicing herbalists. www.AmericanHerbalistsGuild.com

Herbal Academy In my opinion, one of the most comprehensive online herbal courses available. Several levels of skill to choose from. www.TheHerbalAcademy.com

Frontier Herbs This website is a source for any certified organic bulk dried herbs and spices and tea-making supplies. www.FrontierCoOp.com

Jean's Greens Herbal Tea Works and Herbal Essentials is a brick and mortar storefront in Troy, NY, but has an extensive online bulk herb catalog. www.JeansGreens.com

Mountain Rose Herbs This store is based in Eugene, OR, and carries a wide variety of bulk herbs and herbal products for culinary, body care, and craft use. www.MountainRoseHerbs.com

HERB INDEX

RECICE INDEX

INDEX

ACKNOWLEDGMENTS

To my students far and near: Every year, your desire and curiosity refresh my own. Sharing the green world with you inspires my work every single day. Thank you for asking all the right questions and for the many memorable faces you make on your introduction to the bitter taste. I love you all.

To my herbal mentor and friend, David Winston: Over 20 years ago you first introduced me to the "taste of herbs." Your teachings on Ayurvedic, Chinese, and Cherokee medicines opened my heart and mind to the expansive healing potential of herbs. Thank you for continually inspiring me on the green path.

To my friend and herbal mentor, Tina Sams: Our long friendship walking this herbal road, your willingness to share all things herbal, and your laughter have meant the world to me. Thank you also for sharing my name with Callisto Media to write this book. Thank you for always giving me the nudge to write, stretch, and shine.

To my editor, Allison Serrell: Thank you for sharing your extensive expertise with me. Your ability to help me fine-tune and clarify my thoughts—and then polish them one more time—has been most helpful. It was my sincere pleasure to work with you

And finally, to my best friend and soulmate, Joseph: Thank you for smiling at me over cheese, bread, and wine at 9 p.m. more times than I care to admit during this writing process. The universe undoubtedly waited to negotiate my lifelong book dream until you were by my side. Your support and encouragement were essential to its completion. I look forward to stirring an extra pinch of love into every single recipe in this book just for you. Salute!

ABOUT THE AUTHOR

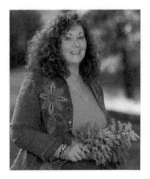 *Susan Hess* is a therapeutic herbalist and native weed wrangler who lives in Mays Landing, New Jersey. She has spent the past 20 years practicing and teaching others about herbs and their uses. Susan teaches an informative 12-month foundation course titled Homestead Herbalism. She enjoys speaking to groups and schools locally on a wide range of herbal topics and is pleased to create an environment that serves to combine community, education, and native and cultivated medicinal plants.

Susan grows a wide variety of medicinal and culinary herbs in her teaching gardens, and she relishes wandering the wild places, discovering native beneficial plants, trees, and mushrooms. She is fully committed to using growing and harvesting methods that protect and replenish the earth and the plants. In her spare time, Susan enjoys researching and studying traditional healing modalities, stargazing, writing, photography, cheesemaking, and stirring up a wide variety of healing foods and herbal creations. For more information about Susan, please visit her website: www.StillRoomatPitchPines.com.